Governors State University
Library
Hours:
Monday thru Thursday 8:30 to 10:30
Friday and Saturday 8:30 to 5:00
Sunday 1:00 to 5:00 (Fall and Winter Trimester Only)

DEMCO

# COMING OUT OF CANCER

*Writings from the*
*Lesbian Cancer Epidemic*

Edited by Victoria A. Brownworth

Seal Press

Cover photograph by Tony Stone
Text design by Alison Rogalsky

Credits appear on page 225, which constitutes a continuation of the copyright page.

*Library of Congress Cataloging-in-Publication Data*

Coming out of cancer: writings from the lesbian cancer epidemic / edited by Victoria A. Brownworth.
  p. cm.
 ISBN 1-58005-044-1 (alk. paper)
 1. Cancer in women. 2. Lesbians—Health and hygiene. I. Brownworth, Victoria A.

RC281.W65 C645 2000
362.1'96994'0082—dc21

                00-056288

Printed in the United States of America

First printing, October 2000

10 9 8 7 6 5 4 3 2 1

Distributed to the trade by Publishers Group West
*In Canada:* Publishers Group West Canada, Toronto, Ontario
*In the U.K. and Europe:* Airlift Book Distributors, Middlesex, England
*In Australia:* Banyan Tree Book Distributors, Kent Town, South Australia

*for the survivors, RR and RLH:*
*to the many anniversaries to come*


*for those who did not survive:*
*that we may fight on, fiercely, in their memory*


*so much depends upon our courage*
*to invent the gestures of survival.*
     —Sandra Steingraber, *Post-Diagnosis*


*To keep our faces toward change and behave like free spirits*
*in the presence of fate is strength undefeatable.*
     —Helen Keller

# Contents

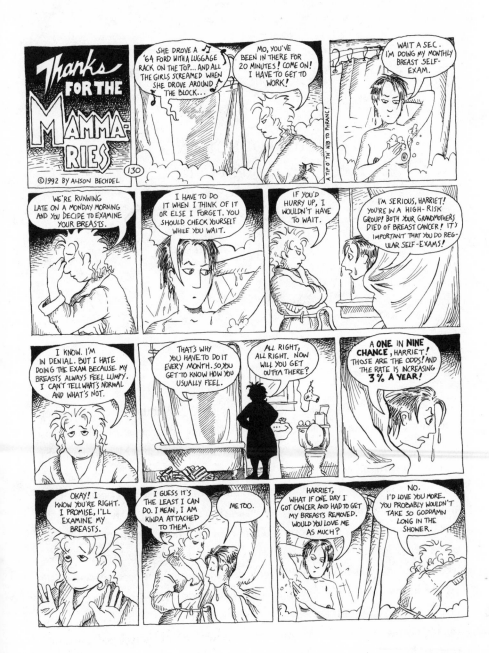

# INTRODUCTION
## A Hidden Cell

*Victoria A. Brownworth*

THE SUN HAD ALREADY BEGUN TO SET on the chill November afternoon when the phone call came. A black thatch of barren tree branches starkly limned an autumn sky riven with color—orange, magenta, purple and blue scarring the horizon beyond my window.

I have received many portentous calls over the past two decades: calls fraught with urgency, calls charged with grief, calls seared with anger—such has been the nature of my work as a reporter, such has been the nature of my queer life. I have covered many stories that could be termed tragic—rapes, assaults, murders. I have spent fifteen years as a medical reporter, covering AIDS: I have stood in hospitals holding babies abandoned because they had AIDS, sat curbside with homeless men and women dying of the disease, investigated hospitals and hospices, interviewed scientists and activists determined to stop the epidemic.

Over the years I have also written extensively about cancer. In the late eighties, I was the first to write about the increased risk of breast cancer lesbians face. I have written about the links between industrial pollution and cancer, about nuclear "accidents," like that of Chernobyl, and the link to cancer. I spent the summer of 1990 investigating the impact of pesticide poisoning on the children of farmworkers in Central California—the hottest summer on record in that state. I have stood at the Superfund sites; gone at dawn to stand under planes illegally dusting not only crops, but also ground water and wells; visited hospital wards filled with children dying of cancers they got from contaminated well water, from houses built on carcinogenic landfill, from playgrounds and schools built flush with fields awash in pesticides; interviewed distraught and disbelieving parents who could not believe that the work they did to provide for their children and the homes they had struggled to buy for their families were the very things killing their children. I was poisoned by pesticides myself that summer; I have been sick ever since.

For two decades I have worked around death—impending death and sudden death—and its disturbing aftermath. Death and I have become so close, I cannot tell if death stalks me or if I stalk it. What I do know is that we always have each other in our sights. And so when the phone call came last November, in the chill afternoon with the sky deep and raw as a wound, I recognized the note of urgency in the voice, the tone of outrage, the slight susurration of grief.

Kathleen DeBold and I had worked together in the past—I as reporter, she as political organizer. The day she called me, she had just assumed the position of executive director of the Mary-Helen Mautner Project for Lesbians with Cancer in Washington, D.C., where the enormity of the cancer epidemic among lesbians had hit her like a body blow. We volleyed names—the famous ones, knowing only too well how many more there were who were unknown—back and forth for some time, and she explained the reason for her call. All these dead lesbians, Kathleen said, and where was the memorial to them and their work? No "Names" quilt, no Capitol Hill testimonies, no national day set aside to address the issue. She voiced concerns that soon the work of certain women might be forgotten, because they were dead and there was no one to stoke the flame of their memory. These women were, I said, a hidden cell, using that old leftist term for its double entendre: the unknown and unrecognized cohort of lesbians with cancer. A hidden cell of women, just like the hidden cell of cancer. And just like the hidden cancer cell can eradicate life, the memories of the hidden cell of lesbians with cancer could be eradicated if no one bore witness to their lives.

Kathleen wanted me to bear witness to those lives with a book—a compilation of work by and about lesbians with cancer, a testimony, a memorial. She wanted the book's publication to coincide with a September 2000 conference on lesbians and cancer sponsored by Mautner.

Years ago an editor of mine told me that books are like babies—it always takes forty weeks to produce one, from manuscript to finished book. And that doesn't include the time it takes to write or research, compile or edit. I told Kathleen it wasn't possible—this was November 1999, after all. But she was adamant that the book be available at the conference and sure that somehow I could make it happen. Decades of activism have taught me that almost nothing is impossible; you can always do more than you think you can. But my own health was fragile, the task Sisyphean. This would be a difficult job for a healthy person—how could I possibly do it? Yet the importance of the project stirred me even as the substance of my conversation with Kathleen resonated. The first woman I had ever lived with had died two weeks earlier from colon cancer, a week after her fiftieth birthday. She was dead, I firmly believed, because her status as a poor, butch lesbian had put the medical care that might have saved her beyond her grasp.

It was a Friday afternoon, the weekend before Thanksgiving. I told Kathleen I would give her an answer Monday, but an hour after our conversation I was talking to a close friend, a lesbian writer with cancer, requisitioning the first piece for the book.

The next few weeks I spent researching—reading massive amounts of essays, poems, fiction, journal entries and memoirs about cancer. A stack of newspaper and magazine clippings began to grow on my bedside table. There was so much cancer. How could I ever write about it all, how could I ever choose enough pieces, the right pieces, the representative pieces of an epidemic that had touched so many women, including myself? How would I get all the ideas I had about lesbians and cancer and what caused the overwhelming epidemic into the book? Could I find the perfect pieces that would detail the sexism, homophobia and racism, the impact of poverty and the environment, the lack of health care, the lack of support—all the things that conspired to target lesbians for cancer? And what about that stack of clippings—the obituaries from Atlanta, Chicago, New York, Philadelphia, Raleigh-Durham and San Francisco torn from the pages of the queer newspapers for which I write; the opinion pieces about cancer scares and cancer survival; the advertisements for local fundraisers for dying women and memorials for women already dead; the short news items about this or that agency proposing to add lesbian cancer concerns to its AIDS agenda or health initiative if funding could be made available? How could I tell the story of each woman whose name had crossed my desk as I compiled material for the book?

There were some voices I immediately knew I had to include—my two best friends, one a writer, one a social worker, both living edgily with the hidden cells of cancer; Pat Parker, poet and activist, whom I had met and interviewed in my earliest days as a reporter and whose presence filled so much space; Rachel Carson, scientist and founder of the environmentalist movement whose transcendent work, *Silent Spring,* had been one of the most memorable books of my youth; Adrienne Rich, whose poem "A Woman Dead in Her Forties" had resonated in my memory since college, more than two decades ago; Joan Nestle, whose chronicles of lesbian life had always moved me. And there would have to be Audre Lorde, who had shown me how one lives with cancer years ago, when I had met her at a party given by friends in New York. Audre had already lost a breast to cancer then and refused to wear a prosthesis. We sat on a sofa together talking, she in a vibrantly printed dashiki and pants, I in a long swirling skirt and a creamy diaphanous blouse revealing a lacy push-up bra. Then the music started and she was up and wanting to dance and pulled me up with her. I will never forget how comfortable she was in her one-breasted amazon body, how she danced as if she hadn't a care in the world, instead of cancer metastasizing through her body, churning through her liver, on the way to killing her.

These were voices that resonated for me.

And soon I found others to complement those. Too many: The retinue of lesbians with cancer was overwhelming. Everyone I spoke to had a cancer story to tell or knew someone who did. So many women, so many different cancers, such divergent experiences of treatment and care and survival—or not. I could not include them all.

Nor was there writing by every lesbian whose voice I wanted memorialized, like Barbara Deming, whose work and philanthropy has so influenced a generation of lesbians. I asked a friend who knew her well if she could write about Barbara's cancer experience. She wrote me a poignant note about how Deming never talked about her cancer, because when she was dying of it, women had yet to break the silence. A few years later, when Deming had already died, Audre broke this silence.

In high school I listened to a range of music from Led Zeppelin to Joni Mitchell to Ella Fitzgerald, but for a year or so I was captivated by Laura Nyro. Her broad hips, long black hair, gypsy dress, sensual mouth and deep, soulful eyes all called out to the romantic in my adolescent lesbian self. Her music was strong, innovative, sensual, introspective; it went through you. In concert she spread herself over the piano as if it were a lover. When Nyro died in 1997 of ovarian cancer at the age of forty-nine, I was shocked. Another lesbian dead. Another special voice silenced.

There are others, of course. Lesbian artist Hollis Sigler attended art school with my friend, Martha Peech, and has been written about extensively by another artist friend, Tee Corinne. In 1999 Sigler shocked the art world that has always embraced her iconoclastic work by declaring not only her lesbianism—still risqué in the tight-fisted world of galleries and curated shows—but also her battle with breast cancer. Her searing documentary of her own experience is *Breast Cancer Journal*, a compilation of the paintings and drawings she has done in recent years detailing her fight for life. Sigler's art reminds some of the daring work of Mexican painter Frida Kahlo, but it has its own singularity. The art in *Breast Cancer Journal* would, Sigler hoped, carry a message: "The work would thus gain the power to destroy the silence surrounding the disease."

I would have liked to have included in this collection the art of Sigler, the music of Nyro and the words never written about cancer by Deming. These women belong here, as do so many others. But it is my hope that in invoking their names, I will send readers forth to investigate their work and to remember what they have created for other women. I hope readers will begin to collect their own cancer stories.

As I write this introduction, the ABC soap opera "One Life to Live" has a breast cancer storyline. A central character in this show that has been on the air for thirty years, fortysomething Viki Carpenter, went for a routine mammogram only to be told the radiologist discovered an "unusual" area on the x-ray. The follow-up tests ensue—ultrasound, biopsy. Each person along the way reminds Viki that the majority of such findings are benign. Her results turn out to be cancer.

Viki undergoes a modified radical mastectomy. Pathology reports indicate that two of the lymph nodes are also involved. The surgery is extensive, the proposed follow-up treatment of radiation and chemotherapy frightening. Erika Slezak, who has played Viki's character for nearly twenty years, has won five Emmys for her performances. She's a fine and nuanced actress and to this story she has brought a slice of reality rarely seen on television, let alone within the heightened unreality of soaps.

Slezak's portrayal of Viki's fear—first when hearing the word cancer, then of losing her breast and possibly her life—has been vivid and, based on my personal experience, quite realistic. The character has gone through the stages of "why me" as well as "what did I do to get this?" After her surgery, rather than having the immediate television recovery, she lay in obvious pain, barely able to speak. As pain lessened and the enormity of what still lay ahead loomed before Viki, a new wave of terror overtook her: fear that she would die, that the ordeal would be too much, that she would not be up to the job of fighting for her own life, just as the thought nagged that she had somehow not been up to the job of preventing herself from getting cancer in the first place. She fears losing her hair, being unable to work, leaning too heavily on her children, having to tell her colleagues and friends despite being a very private person who doesn't share such intimate details readily.

A newspaper editor, Viki begins recording her experience on her laptop computer. A few days after her surgery, she lies in her hospital bed typing out these thoughts—with one hand because the surgerized side is too painful and damaged to use yet—because she believes somehow it will give her strength to record her experience.

Viki's surgeon, a woman, tells her the operation was quite successful.

Reconstruction was done and the surgeon tells Viki she will look perfectly normal in clothes. Viki and the audience hear the distinction. In clothes—not naked. This will be no perfect television plastic surgery.

When Viki goes home from the hospital again, there is no miracle soap-style/romanticized television version of cancer. She sits, weak, with her left arm on a pillow—still feeling intense pain from the surgery. A few days later she asks her surgeon to help her view the breast that has been cut away and then reconstructed. Viki has yet to look at what lies beneath the bandages. The audience sees her as she looks in the mirror, the range of emotion on her face—shock, revulsion, pain. "It's not me," she says softly.

Days later Viki also does what many women facing chemotherapy do: She has her hair cut very short in an attempt to lessen the shock of hair loss that accompanies chemotherapy and to take control of the situation as much as she can.

Ten years ago this would not have been a storyline on a soap opera—too grim, too realistic, too much like the lives of the women watching the soap as they tend small children, work at home, recover from illnesses. The number of women coping with cancer has surged so dramatically that even the romantic world of soaps has begun to address the issue.

The significance of this cannot be overstated—nor can this particular portrayal. This major character will not be killed off, nor, however, is she going to get a medical slap on the wrist. Viki will not have, as they say, a surgical resolution. She will, as do the majority of women who undergo modified radical mastectomies, endure months of radiation and chemotherapy and with those grueling treatments the added assaults of nausea, hair loss, weight gain and incomparable fatigue. She will look in the mirror and not always recognize herself. She will wonder again and again if she can survive this treatment that will allegedly restore her to her precancerous state—minus the breast she once had and the hair and the svelte shape and the boundless energy. She will wonder—because she cannot help but do so—*why* she got this cancer and *how* she got it.

The issue of representation—accurate representation—of cancer arises again and again. Yet there remains a certain proscription against accuracy. Too grim, inevitably. Ruthann Robson's essay in this collection addresses this point: We shared an almost exact experience, nearly word for word, of being told when pitching cancer stories to editors, that cancer isn't—as I was told—"sexy." Nevertheless, the drama of cancer inevitably finds its way—inaccurately—into fiction and film and television and all the avenues popular culture traverses.

When it became clear that AIDS would not be a short-lived virus but a long-term scourge upon the queer landscape, writers began to record their experiences—as people with AIDS, as friends of the dying, as activists. In the first decade of the AIDS pandemic the link between gay men and AIDS was so internecine—and so seemingly irrevocable—that the body of literature that evolved was as much queer as it was about AIDS. Now we know that AIDS kills with little concern for sexual orientation or gender or age or race or environment. AIDS, we have come to say, is an equal-opportunity killer.

Similarly cancer always appeared to strike its victims randomly. We came to know the smokers would get it—lung, throat, stomach, mouth—there was little likelihood of escape. But the other victims seemed chosen at random—children with leukemia and eye cancer, women with breast and gynecological cancers, men with prostate cancer, everyone with colon and skin cancer, young adults with Hodgkins and melanoma, older people with brain and liver cancer. Where was the connection? Thus an inevitability in how lesbians were slow to accept their own heightened risk seemed natural. The lack of representation derived more from fear than ignorance—if you don't write it down, it won't be real. But in not writing about our experiences of cancer, we have left a void.

As I reread Audre Lorde's cancer journals, trying to decide which entries to choose for this collection, I was so moved and struck by her words—the depth and sincerity, the determination, the activism, the refusal to ignore her own privileged status despite being a black lesbian in a straight white country. Her words had such impact, reminding me of why I do the work I do and what it means to be an activist in an increasingly apathetic, status quo–oriented culture.

Thus I focused on representation as the most essential aspect of this collection. Certainly I needed to address race—that was a given. But I also needed to address class and privilege and how it altered care and survival. I needed to address the range of cancer experiences because breast cancer is not the only cancer lesbians endure. My two closest friends, for example, were diagnosed with rare cancers. And what about lung cancer? Lung cancer victims have come to be treated the way adults with AIDS were treated in the early years of the pandemic. As if there are "innocent" victims of disease and those who are implicated in their own mortality. In reading the interview with Vivian Kasper about the death of her lover of more than thirty years, the impact of smoking on generations of women cannot be dismissed. Even as she lay in the hospital, Rose begged her lover Vivian for a cigarette.

One of the new trends in medicine—even alternative treatments—is to implicate the patient in her disease and recovery. Type A personalities (of which I am one) are prone to cancer. Workaholics (of which I am one) are prone to cancer. Internalized anger predisposes one to cancer as do unresolved feelings. And then there is diet and exercise and lifestyle and . . . the list goes on. "Curing" one's self presents another daunting responsibility. Seek a range of treatments, creatively visualize cancer cells leaving the body, imagine blue and violet light because these are the healing end of the spectrum and so on. Therefore, if lesbians know they are at heightened risk for cancer, aren't they responsible for that fact in some way?

In 1995 my favorite cat, Magda, died of liver cancer. She was old—over sixteen—and the vet told me all animals die of cancer if they live long enough. Magda had died only three weeks after my lover's and my dog Coco, also sixteen, had died of a massive, inoperable tumor that ran from the back of her throat into her chest. The words of the vet echoed for months—*all animals die of cancer if they live long enough*.

It was Rachel Carson who first began to make the connection between our environment and our bodies and the larger body of the planet. What we do to the environment would, she cautioned, come back to haunt us and perhaps kill us. Her admonitions have gone unheeded. Each day carcinogenic material is spewed into the air, water and earth. Last week I listened to a conservative lobbyist argue on the television talk show *Politically Incorrect* that we should adopt a "wait and see" approach to global warming and toxic air and water. He explained that developing countries need to strip the rain forests while global corporations must be allowed to expand production. On the same panel was Julia Butterfly Hill, a woman who spent two years living in a tree to keep it from being cut down. When the conservative challenged her on her comments that trees spoke to her, the activist said, "You can attempt to discredit me by taking my words out of context and trivializing the way I have spent the last two years of my life. But the planet as a whole is trying to tell us something: that we are killing it and us, and we must stop." How much cancer is caused by growth hormones in milk and poultry, by DDT and other pesticides lurking first in the environment and then in the soft tissue of women, by the gases that spew out of cars and factories and energy plants, by the radiation that emanates from televisions, computers, cell phones, electric towers? These are questions that have yet to be answered.

When I was researching the pesticide series among the farmworkers in California, the photographer from the newspaper with whom I was traveling, David Wells, remarked one night over dinner that it was the consumer's lust for the perfect fruit and vegetable—unblemished by weevil spots or snail tracks or wormholes—that was killing the children of the San Joaquin Valley. David's sister and brother-in-law were nurses at the hospital in Fresno where the children's cancer ward was five times the size of the one in our own city, Philadelphia, the nation's fifth largest city.

As we traveled hundreds of miles each day to small towns that formed the web of California's Central Valley, we drove through acres and acres of perfect croplands—impossibly green fields of cotton, soybeans and strawberries, multihued carpets of carnations and roses (California is the largest producer of these flowers in the world), densely packed arbors of grapes and thick orchards of lime, lemon, peach and almond trees. The verdant landscape offset by unrelieved sunshine and a cinematically perfect azure sky belied the pesticide warnings in the signs reading *peligro*—danger—at the entrance to one or another row of crops.

One day I yelled at David to stop the car. I wanted him to take a picture. Photographers don't view themselves as adjuncts to reporters, and he balked at my directive—until he saw the scene I had caught peripherally as we sped down the highway. A group of children—none older than seven—played with action figures in a small waterhole at the edge of an almond grove. It was an intolerably hot day—the heat was searing—and the waterhole gave off a wisp of coolness, shaded as it was by the almond trees.

But the water wasn't a place for play; it was pesticide runoff from the cotton field angled across from the orchard. I had seen the little red skull and crossbones stark against the white cardboard sign positioned at the perimeter of the hole. I had almost heard rather than read *peligro*, big and bold below the international sign for death. But these children—unsupervised, as their parents no doubt worked in the hot depths of the fields beyond—saw no sign, read no warning, intuited nothing from the milky sheen upon the water save their own desire for play and some small relief from the heat.


*All animals die from cancer if they live long enough.* Or sooner, if they are like the canaries in the mines—the frogs worldwide being born anomalous and freakish from contaminated water, dying at an alarming rate; the birds clustered in little carrion piles at the mouths of tributaries near pesticide-laden fields or industrial parks.

I have come to view lesbians as Darwinian test cases as well—the queer canaries in the cancer mine of the twenty-first century. Our desire for connection with other lesbians leads us to urban areas (the three major queer meccas in America—New York, Los Angeles and San Francisco—also house the top two cancer vectors), where our lower economic and class status make us less likely to be able to get jobs or housing in places untainted by environmental pollutants. Our experiences with sexism, homophobia and racism make it less likely for us to seek out medical care, even when we need it, though our precarious financial status often precludes our ability to pay for such services regardless. We are second-class citizens and our cancer rates reflect that status.

When I first wrote about the heightened risk for breast cancer among lesbians early in 1993 for *Out* magazine, Audre Lorde had just died and a little-known researcher at the National Cancer Institute, Dr. Suzanne Haynes, had recently published a small study. She suggested that although the breast cancer risk for women overall was one in nine (it became one in eight a year later), the risk for lesbians was a startling one in three. As I interviewed lesbians across the country for the article, I was stunned by how many had cancer and how many had experienced shoddy and homophobic care. Meanwhile, there were no support services for lesbians with cancer either—and as one woman explained, the concerns of a straight woman about her husband's response to her missing breast were very different from the concerns of lesbians about coming out to their doctors.

In compiling this collection, I found, regrettably, that little had changed in the intervening years since I wrote that piece. So little that I had intended to add it to this collection, but then decided this book would speak to that issue itself, through the words of pioneering surgeon and activist Dr. Susan Love, through Lynn Kanter's history of lesbian cancer activism, through Paula Berg's explication of how to get essential medical care and through the fact that the Mautner Project, the nation's oldest cancer organization for lesbians, had requisitioned this book in the first place.

Still, this anthology is meant to be a historical document, and so I wanted to include pieces that would resonate back to a time before we spoke of these things, before we ever considered that we might be test cases or that we might be able to step out into the light and declare both our lesbianism and our cancer status and demand equal treatment for both. Adrienne Rich writes in her poem, "A Woman Dead in Her Forties," "but we never spoke of such things," a line that, although it references sexuality in the poem, deftly sums up the years in which silence determined how lesbians dealt with the enormity of cancer.

The length of this insidious epidemic is as awesome as it is terrible. As I worked on this book, I talked with several women much my junior—lesbians in their twenties. Political lesbians, well-read lesbians but women young enough to be my daughters, women of an entirely different generation. And I found Kathleen DeBold's fears had been confirmed: The names of the casualties in this war have already faded from memory. These lesbians have heard the name Pat Parker but are unfamiliar with her work. None had ever heard of Jackie Winnow. None knew Rachel Carson had died so young—because these days, fifty-one is young—of cancer.

Enough time has passed that Sandra Steingraber—whose work as a biologist, environmentalist and writer has led her down the path first hewn a generation earlier by Rachel Carson—has uncovered that new generation's hideous secrets: in nuclear waste and in industrial accidents and in her own body. Enough time has passed that Teya Schaffer, who still mourns the death of her lover, Jackie Winnow, has watched her child grow up—another generation. Enough time has passed that I am now the age Audre Lorde was when she was diagnosed with breast cancer. Enough time has passed that we are in terrible peril of forgetting just how much we have lost to cancer because we continue to lose so much more. In this graveyard the inscriptions have already begun to wear away even as new deaths toll daily.

The uplifting title of this anthology belies much of what lies between these covers; cancer leaves few happy endings. There are the voices of the dead and the voices of their loved ones who fan the flames of memory, light the *yahrzeit* candles to remind us they were once here. There are also the voices of survivors—some perhaps just clinging to life; others far more sure they have been cured; still others walking that uneasy line between tests and follow-ups. What lies between these book covers is testimony and testament—witness borne to a war against a hidden cell, cancer, by that other hidden cell, the lesbian cancer cohort. What lies between these covers is representative of the lesbian cancer experience, broad though that experience may be. What lies between these covers is grief and anger and despair and hope. What lies between these covers is a history of who we were, are and will be—our past, present and determined struggle to survive into the future.

*Victoria A. Brownworth*
*Philadelphia*
*May 2000*

# COMING OUT OF CANCER

# A Burst of Light
## Living with Cancer

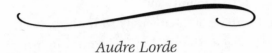

*Audre Lorde*

*though we may land here there is no other landing*
*to choose our meaning we must make it new.*
Muriel Rukeyser

## Introduction

The year I became fifty felt like a great coming together for me. I was very proud of having made it for half a century, and in my own style. "Time for a change," I thought, "I wonder how I'm going to live the next half."

On February 1st, two weeks before my fiftieth birthday, I was told by my doctor that I had liver cancer, metastasized from the breast cancer for which I had had a mastectomy six years before.

At first I did not believe it. I continued with my previously planned teaching trip to Europe. As I grew steadily sicker in Berlin, I received medical information about homeopathic alternatives to surgery, which strengthened my decision to maintain some control over my life for as long as possible. I believe that decision has prolonged my life, together with the loving energies of women who supported me in that decision and in the work which gives that life shape.

The struggle with cancer now informs all my days, but it is only another face of that continuing battle for self-determination and survival that Black women fight daily, often in triumph. The following excerpts are from journals kept during my first three years of living with cancer.

## March 18, 1984
### En route to St. Croix, Virgin Islands

I've written nothing of the intensity with which I've lived the last few weeks. The hepatologist who tried to frighten me into an immediate liver biopsy without even listening to my objections and questions. Seeing the growth in my liver on the CAT scan, doing a face-off with death, again. Not again, just escalated. This mass in my liver is not a primary liver tumor, so if it is malignant, it's most likely metastasized breast cancer. Not curable. Arrestable, not curable. This is a very bad dream, and I'm the only person who can wake myself up. I had a talk before I left with Peter, my breast surgeon. He says that if it is liver cancer, with the standard treatments—surgery, radiation, and chemotherapy—we're talking four or five years at best. Without treatment, he says, maybe three or four.

In other words, western medicine doesn't have a very impressive track record with cancer metastasized to the liver.

In the light of those facts, and from all the reading I've been doing these past weeks (thank the goddess for Barnes & Noble's Medical Section), I've made up my mind not to have a liver biopsy. It feels like the only reasonable decision for me. I'm asymptomatic now except for a vicious gallbladder. And I can placate her. There are too many things I'm determined to do that I haven't done yet. Finish the poem "Outlines." See what Europe's all about. Make Deotha Chamber's story live.

If I have this biopsy and it is malignant, then a whole course of action will be established simply by their intrusion into the suspect site. Yet if this tumor is malignant, I want as much good time as possible, and their treatments aren't going to make a hell of a lot of difference in terms of extended time. But they'll make a hell of a lot of difference in terms of my general condition and how I live my life.

On the other hand, if this is benign, I believe surgical intervention into fatty tissue of any kind can start the malignant process in what otherwise might remain benign for a long time. I've been down that road before.

I've decided this is a chance I have to take. If this were another breast tumor, I'd go for surgery again, because the organ comes off. But with the tie-in between estrogens, fat cells, and malignancies I've been reading about, cutting into my liver seems to me to be too much of a risk for too little return in terms of time. And it might be benign, some little aberrant joke between my liver and the universe.

Twenty-two hours of most days I don't believe I have liver cancer. Most days. Those other two hours of the day are pure hell, and there's so much work I have to do in my head in those two hours, too, through all the terror and uncertainties.

I wish I knew a doctor I could really trust to talk it all over with. Am I making the right decision? I know I have to listen to my body. If there's one thing I've learned from all the work I've done since my mastectomy, it's that I must listen keenly to the messages my body sends. But sometimes they are contradictory.

Dear goddess! Face-up again against the renewal of vows. Do not let me die a coward, mother. Nor forget how to sing. Nor forget song is a part of mourning as light is a part of sun.

## June 1, 1984
## Berlin

My classes are exciting and exhausting. Black women are hearing about them and their number is increasing.

I can't eat cooked food and I am getting sicker. My liver is so swollen I can feel it under my ribs. I've lost almost fifty pounds. That's a switch, worrying about losing weight. My friend Dagmar, who teaches here, has given me the name of a homeopathic doctor specializing in the treatment of cancer, and I've made an appointment to see her when I come back from the Feminist Bookfair in London next week. She's an anthroposophic doctor, and they believe in surgery only as a last resort.

In spite of all this, I'm doing good work here. I'm certainly enjoying life in Berlin, sick or not. The city itself is very different from what I'd expected. It is lively and beautiful, but its past is never very far away, at least not for me. The silence about Jews is absolutely deafening, chilling. There is only one memorial in the whole city and it is to the Resistance. At the entrance is a huge grey urn with the sign, "This urn contains earth from German concentration camps." It is such a euphemistic evasion of responsibility and an invitation to amnesia for the children that it's no wonder my students act like Nazism was a bad dream not to be remembered.

There is a lot of networking going on here among women, collectives and work enterprises as well as political initiatives, and a very active women's cultural scene. I may be too thin, but I can still dance!

**June 7, 1984**
**Berlin**

Dr. Rosenberg agrees with my decision not to have a biopsy, but she has said I must do something quickly to strengthen my bodily defenses. She's recommended I begin Iscador injections three times weekly.

Iscador is a biological made from mistletoe which strengthens the natural immune system, and works against the growth of malignant cells. I've started the injections, along with two other herbals that stimulate liver function. I feel less weak.

I am listening to what fear teaches. I will never be gone. I am a scar, a report from the frontlines, a talisman, a resurrection. A rough place on the chin of complacency. "What are you getting so upset about, anyway?" a student asked in class, "You're not Jewish!"

So what if I am afraid? Of stepping out into the morning? Of dying? Of unleashing the damned gall where hatred swims like a tadpole waiting to swell into the arms of war? And what does that war teach when the bruised leavings jump an insurmountable wall where the glorious Berlin chestnuts and orange poppies hide detection wires that spray bullets which kill?

My poems are filled with blood these days because the future is so bloody. When the blood of four-year-old children runs unremarked through the alleys of Soweto, how can I pretend that sweetness is anything more than armor and ammunition in an on-going war?

I am saving my life by using my life in the service of what must be done. Tonight as I listened to the ANC speakers from South Africa at the Third World People's Center here, I was filled with a sense of self answering necessity, of commitment as a survival weapon. Our battles are inseparable. Every person I have ever been must be actively enlisted in those battles, as well as in the battle to save my life.

## June 9, 1984
## Berlin

At the poetry reading in Zurich this weekend, I found it so much easier to discuss racism than to talk about *The Cancer Journals*. Chemical plants between Zurich and Basel have been implicated in a definite rise in breast cancer in this region, and women wanted to discuss this. I talked as honestly as I could, but it was really hard. Their questions presume a clarity I no longer have.

It was great to have Gloria there to help field all those questions about racism. For the first time in Europe, I felt I was not alone but answering as one of a group of Black women—not just Audre Lorde!

I am cultivating every iota of my energies to do battle with the possibility of liver cancer. At the same time, I am discovering how furious and resistant some pieces of me are, as well as how terrified.

In this loneliest of places, I examine every decision I make within the light of what I've learned about myself and that self-destructiveness implanted inside of me by racism and sexism and the circumstances of my life as a Black woman.

*Mother why were we armed to fight*
*with cloud wreathed swords and javelins of dust?*

Survival isn't some theory operating in a vacuum. It's a matter of my everyday living and making decisions.

How do I hold faith with sun in a sunless place? It is so hard not to counter this despair with a refusal to see. But I have to stay open and filtering no matter what's coming at me, because that arms me in a particularly Black woman's way. When I'm open, I'm also less despairing. The more clearly I see what I'm up against, the more able I am to fight this process going on in my body that they're calling liver cancer. And I am determined to fight it even when I am not sure of the terms of the battle nor the face of victory. I just know I must not surrender my body to others unless I completely understand and agree with what they think should be done to it. I've got to look at all of my options carefully, even the ones I find distasteful. I know I can broaden the definition of winning to the point where I can't lose.

## June 10, 1984
## Berlin

Dr. Rosenberg is honest, straightforward, and pretty discouraging. I don't know what I'd do without Dagmar there to translate all her grim pronouncements for me. She thinks it's liver cancer, too, but she respects my decision against surgery. I mustn't let my unwillingness to accept this diagnosis interfere with getting help. Whatever it is, this seems to be working.

We all have to die at least once. Making that death useful would be winning for me. I wasn't supposed to exist anyway, not in any meaningful way in this fucked-up whiteboys' world. I want desperately to live, and I'm ready to fight for that living even if I die shortly. Just writing those words down snaps every thing I want to do into a neon clarity. This European trip and the Afro-German women, the Sister Outsider collective in Holland, Gloria's great idea of starting an organization that can be a connection between us and South African women. For the first time I really feel that my writing has a substance and stature that will survive me.

I have done good work. I see it in the letters that come to me about *Sister Outsider*, I see it in the use the women here give the poetry and the prose. But first and last I am a poet. I've worked very hard for that approach to living inside myself, and everything I do, I hope, reflects that view of life, even the ways I must move now in order to save my life.

I have done good work. There is a hell of a lot more I have to do. And sitting here tonight in this lovely green park in Berlin, dusk approaching and the walking willows leaning over the edge of the pool caressing each other's fingers, birds birds birds singing under and over the frogs, and the smell of new-mown grass enveloping my sad pen, I feel I still have enough moxie to do it all, on whatever terms I'm dealt, timely or not. Enough moxie to chew the whole world up and spit it out in bite-sized pieces, useful and warm and wet and delectable because they came out of my mouth.

## November 21, 1985
## New York City

It feels like the axe is falling. There it is on the new CAT scan—another mass growing in my liver, and the first one is spreading. I've found an anthroposophic doctor in Spring Valley who suggests I go to the Lukas Klinik, a hospital in Switzerland where they are conducting the primary research on Iscador, as well as diagnosing and treating cancers.

I've known something is wrong from the returning pains and the dimming energies of my body. My classes have been difficult, and most days I feel like I'm going on sheer will power alone which can be very freeing and seductive but also very dangerous. Limited. I'm running down. But I'd do exactly what I'm doing anyway, cancer or no cancer.

A. will lend us the money to go to Switzerland, and Frances will come with me. I think they will be able to find out what is really wrong with me at the Lukas Klinik, and if they say these growths in my liver are malignant, then I will accept that I have cancer of the liver. At least there they will be able to adjust my Iscador dosage upward to the maximum effect, because that is the way I have decided to go and I'm not going to change now. Obviously, I still don't accept these tumors in my liver as cancer, although I know that could just be denial on my part, which is certainly one mechanism for coping with cancer. I have to consider denial as a possibility in all of my planning, but I also feel that there is absolutely nothing they can do for me at Sloan-Kettering except cut me open and then sew me back up with their condemnations inside me.

## December 7, 1985
## New York City

My stomach x-rays are clear, and the problems in my GI series are all circumstantial. Now that the doctors here have decided I have liver cancer, they insist on reading all their findings as if that were a *fait accompli*. They refuse to look for any other reason for the irregularities in the x-rays, and they're treating my resistance to their diagnosis as a personal affront. But it's my body and my life and the goddess knows I'm paying enough for all this, I ought to have a say.

The flame is very dim these days. It's all I can do to teach my classes at Hunter and crawl home. Frances and I will leave for Switzerland as soon as school is over next week. The Women's Poetry Center will be dedicated at Hunter the night before I leave. No matter how sick I feel, I'm still afire with a need to do something for my living. How will I be allowed to live my own life, the rest of my life?

## November 8, 1986
## New York City

If I am to put this all down in a way that is useful, I should start with the beginning of the story.

Sizable tumor in the right lobe of the liver, the doctors said. Lots of blood vessels in it means it's most likely malignant. Let's cut you open right now and see what we can do about it. Wait a minute, I said. I need to feel this thing out and see what's going on inside myself first, I said, needing some time to absorb the shock, time to assay the situation and not act out of panic. Not one of them said, I can respect that, but don't take too long about it.

Instead, that simple claim to my body's own processes elicited such an attack response from a reputable Specialist In Liver Tumors that my deepest—if not necessarily most useful—suspicions were totally aroused.

What that doctor could have said to me that I would have heard was, "You have a serious condition going on in your body and whatever you do about it you must not ignore it or delay deciding how you are going to deal with it because it will not go away no matter what you think it is." Acknowledging my responsibility for my own body. Instead, what he said to me was, "If you do not do exactly what I tell you to do right now without questions you are going to die a horrible death." In exactly those words.

I felt the battle lines being drawn up within my own body.

I saw this specialist in liver tumors at a leading cancer hospital in New

York City, where I had been referred as an outpatient by my own doctor.

The first people who interviewed me in white coats from behind a computer were only interested in my health-care benefits and proposed method of payment. Those crucial facts determined what kind of plastic ID card I would be given, and without a plastic ID card, no one at all was allowed upstairs to see any doctor, as I was told by the uniformed, pistoled guards at all the stairwells.

From the moment I was ushered into the doctor's office and he saw my x-rays, he proceeded to infantalize me with an obviously well-practiced technique. When I told him I was having second thoughts about a liver biopsy, he glanced at my chart. Racism and Sexism joined hands across his table as he saw I taught at a university. "Well, you look like an *intelligent girl*," he said, staring at my one breast all the time he was speaking. "Not to have this biopsy immediately is like sticking your head in the sand." Then he went on to say that he would not be responsible when I wound up one day screaming in agony in the corner of his office!

I asked this specialist in liver tumors about the dangers of a liver biopsy spreading an existing malignancy, or even encouraging it in a borderline tumor. He dismissed my concerns with a wave of his hand, saying, instead of answering, that I really did not have any other sensible choice.

I would like to think that this doctor was sincerely motivated by a desire for me to seek what he truly believed to be the only remedy for my sickening body, but my faith in that scenario is considerably diminished by his $250 consultation fee and his subsequent medical report to my own doctor containing numerous supposedly clinical observations of *obese abdomen* and *remaining pendulous breast*.

In any event, I can thank him for the fierce shard lancing through my terror that shrieked there must be some other way, this doesn't feel right to me. If this is cancer and they cut me open to find out, what is stopping that intrusive action from spreading the cancer, or turning a questionable mass into an active malignancy? All I was asking for was the reassurance of a realistic answer to my real questions, and that was not forthcoming. I made up my mind that if I was going to die in agony on somebody's office floor, it certainly wasn't going to be his! I needed information, and pored over books on the liver in Barnes & Noble's Medical Textbook Section on Fifth Avenue for hours. I learned, among other things, that the liver is the largest, most complex, and most generous organ in the human body. But that did not help me very much.

In this period of physical weakness and psychic turmoil, I found myself going through an intricate inventory of rage. First of all at my breast surgeon— had he perhaps done something wrong? How could such a small breast tumor have metastasized? Hadn't he assured me he'd gotten it all, and what was this now anyway about micro-metastases? Could this tumor in my liver have been seeded at the same time as my breast cancer? There were so many unanswered questions, and too much that I just did not understand.

But my worst rage was the rage at myself. For a brief time I felt like a total failure. What had I been busting my ass doing these past six years if it wasn't living and loving and working to my utmost potential? And wasn't that all a guarantee supposed to keep exactly this kind of thing from ever happening again? So what had I done wrong and what was I going to have to pay for it and WHY ME?

But finally a little voice inside me said sharply, "Now really, is there any other way you would have preferred living the past six years that would have been more satisfying? And be that as it may, *should* or *shouldn't* isn't even the question. How do you want to live the rest of your life from now on and what are you going to do about it?" Time's awasting!

Gradually, in those hours in the stacks of Barnes & Noble, I felt myself shifting into another gear. My resolve strengthened as my panic lessened. Deep breathing, regularly. I'm not going to let them cut into my body again until I'm convinced there is no other alternative. And this time, the burden of proof rests with the doctors because their record of success with liver cancer is not so good that it would make me jump at a surgical solution. And scare tactics are not going to work. I have been scared now for six years and that hasn't stopped me. I've given myself plenty of practice in doing whatever I need to do, scared or not, so scare tactics are just not going to work. Or I hoped they were not going to work. At any rate, thank the goddess, they were not working yet. One step at a time.

But some of my nightmares were pure hell, and I started having trouble sleeping.

In writing this I have discovered how important some things are that I thought were unimportant. I discovered this by the high price they exact for scrutiny. At first I did not want to look again at how I slowly came to terms with my own mortality on a level deeper than before, nor with the inevitable strength that gave me as I started to get on with my life in actual time. Medical textbooks on the liver were fine, but there were appointments to be kept, and bills to pay, and decisions about my upcoming trip to Europe to be made. And what do I say to my children? Honesty has always been the bottom line between us, but did I really need them going through this with me during their final difficult years at college? On the other hand, how could I shut them out of this most important decision of my life?

I made a visit to my breast surgeon, a doctor with whom I have always been able to talk frankly, and it was from him that I got my first trustworthy and objective sense of timing. It was from him that I learned that the conventional forms of treatment for liver metastases made little more than one year's difference in the survival rate. I heard my old friend Clem's voice coming back to me through the dimness of thirty years: "I see you coming here trying to make sense where there is no sense. Try just living in it. Respond, alter, see what happens." I thought of the African way of perceiving life, as experience to be lived rather than as problem to be solved.

Homeopathic medicine calls cancer the cold disease. I understand that down to my bones that quake sometimes in their need for heat, for the sun, even for just a hot bath. Part of the way in which I am saving my own life is to refuse to submit my body to cold whenever possible.

In general, I fight hard to keep my treatment scene together in some coherent and serviceable way, integrated into my daily living and absolute. Forgetting is no excuse. It's as simple as one missed shot could make the difference between a quiescent malignancy and one that is growing again. This not only keeps me in an intimate, positive relationship to my own health, but it also underlines the fact that I have the responsibility for attending my own health. I cannot simply hand over that responsibility to anybody else.

Which does not mean I give in to the belief, arrogant or naive, that I know everything I need to know in order to make informed decisions about my body. But attending my own health, gaining enough information to help me understand and participate in the decisions made about my body by people who know more medicine than I do, are all crucial strategies in my battle for living. They also provide me with important prototypes for doing battle in all other arenas of my life.

Battling racism and battling heterosexism and battling apartheid share the same urgency inside me as battling cancer. None of these struggles are ever easy, and even the smallest victory is never to be taken for granted. Each victory must be applauded, because it is so easy not to battle at all, to just accept and call that acceptance inevitable.

And all power is relative. Recognizing the existence as well as the limitations of my own power, and accepting the responsibility for using it in my own behalf, involve me in direct and daily actions that preclude denial as a possible refuge. Simone de Beauvoir's words echo in my head: "It is in the recognition of the genuine conditions of our lives that we gain the strength to act and our motivation for change."

**November 17, 1986**
**New York City**

How has everyday living changed for me with the advent of a second cancer? I move through a terrible and invigorating savor of now—a visceral awareness of the passage of time, with its nightmare and its energy. No more long-term loans, extended payments, twenty-year plans. Pay my debts. Call the tickets in, the charges, the emotional IOU's. Now is the time, if ever, once and for all, to alter the patterns of isolation. Remember that nice lady down the street whose son you used to cross at the light and who was always saying, "Now if there's ever anything I can do for you, just let me know." Well, her boy's got strong muscles and the lawn needs mowing.

I am not ashamed to let my friends know I need their collective spirit— not to make me live forever, but rather to help me move through the life I have. But I refuse to spend the rest of that life mourning what I do not have.

If living as a poet—living on the front lines—has ever had meaning, it has meaning now. Living a self-conscious life, vulnerability as armor.

I spend time every day meditating upon my physical self in battle, visualizing the actual war going on inside my body. As I move through the other parts of each day, that battle often merges with particular external campaigns, both political and personal. The devastations of apartheid in South Africa and racial murder in Howard Beach feel as critical to me as cancer.

Among my other daily activities I incorporate brief periods of physical self-monitoring without hysteria. I attend the changes within my body, anointing myself with healing light. Sometimes I have to do it while sitting on the Staten Island Ferry on my way home, surrounded by snapping gum and dirty rubber boots, all of which I banish from my consciousness.

I am learning to reduce stress in my practical everyday living. It's nonsense, however, to believe that any Black woman who is living an informed life in america can possibly abolish stress totally from her life without becoming psychically deaf, mute, and blind. (*News Item: Unidentified Black man found hanging from a tree in Central Park with hands and feet bound. New York City police call it a suicide.*) I am learning to balance stress with periods of rest and restoration.

I juggle the technologies of eastern medicine with the holistic approach of anthroposophy with the richness of my psychic life, beautifully and womanfully nourished by people I love and who love me. Balancing them all. Knowing over and over again how blessed I am in my life, my loves, my children; how blessed I am in being able to give myself to work in which I passionately believe. And yes, some days I wish to heaven to Mawu to Seboulisa to Tiamat daughter of chaos that it could all have been easier.

But I wake in an early morning to see the sun rise over the tenements of Brooklyn across the bay, fingering through the wintered arms of the raintree Frances and I planted as a thin stick seventeen years ago, and I cannot possibly imagine trading my life for anyone else's, no matter how near termination that life may be. Living fully—how long is not the point. How and why take total precedence.

## December 7, 1986
## New York City

I'm glad I don't have to turn away any more from movies about people dying of cancer. I no longer have to deny cancer as a reality in my life. As I wept over *Terms Of Endearment* last night, I also laughed. It's hard to believe I avoided this movie for over two years.

Yet while I was watching it, involved in the situation of a young mother dying of breast cancer, I was also very aware of that standard of living, taken for granted in the film, that made the expression of her tragedy possible. Her mother's maid and the manicured garden, the unremarked but very tangible money so evident through its effects. Daughter's philandering husband is an unsuccessful English professor, but they still live in a white-shingled house with trees, not in some rack-ass tenement on the Lower East Side or in Harlem for which they pay too much rent.

Her private room in Lincoln Memorial Hospital has her mama's Renoir on the wall. There are never any Black people at all visible in that hospital in Lincoln, Nebraska, not even in the background. Now this may not make her death scenes any less touching, but it did strengthen my resolve to talk about my experiences with breast cancer as a Black woman.

# Apology to Audre Lorde, Never Sent

*Sandra Steingraber*

YEARS LATER, SHE CAME TO MY UNIVERSITY to speak. She said all the beautiful things: about the master's tools and the master's house, about learning to speak when we are afraid. In the back of the auditorium, I wanted my brain to be a tape recorder, a programmed VCR. I wanted my head to be a magnetic tape so that my soul could fly out to where it was already flying, flying to the space with no name, the space that is absence, the space where the cloth folds along her chest, the phantom, amputated space, smooth and broad, a site of violence that she will not hide or reconstruct. I wanted to fall into that emptiness. I was falling, like into tall grass that has grown over war and is peace. I was falling, as though to lie and sleep, curled along her scar like a river.

Please, do not romanticize this. Surely, this is pornography. Come back, my soul, you cannot go there.

Oh Audre, I heard you've had news of a recent metastasis. I want to tell you about my mother's paper towel breasts, how they felt against my ribs when she embraced me. Paper towels, like she's trying to mop up a little accident. Soak up spilled milk she won't cry over, she says, handing me her copies of

Norman Vincent Peale, Helen Steiner Rice, all her three-named authors whose books I broke windows with. Anger purifies. Audre, I want to tell you about the catheter tube that stretched between my own two legs, how I still reach for it in my sleep, that horrible penis. Your words saved me. I was yoked to terrible things then. So, during the questions and answers, I did stand up in that auditorium, shaking like I am now, to say thank you. To say that I had jumped the barrier myself and was saved now. Afterward, in the wine and cheese room, I was embarrassed, I averted my gaze. And then someone nudged me, whispered, "She wants you." And unbelievingly I looked and saw her smiling and beckoning to me as from a distant shore, motioning me to sit down beside her. And I began swimming against an immense current, passing the long snake of people queued before her for book signing.

Oh, Audre. My mother's paper towel breasts pressing my own. It hurt so much. And then me, and everyone thinking it's genetic, but it's not, you know. I was an adopted child, another story, not mine, unremembered, before language. But I memorized your words: "The idea that happiness can insulate us against the results of our environmental madness is a rumor circulated by our enemies to destroy us."[1] The world's largest trash incinerator is going on line in Detroit, and by their own admission, it will raise the cancer rate here. Who speaks for the air and the water? I want to. Oh, Audre, let's leave this hall and walk to the hospital together. We can stroll along the Huron River[2] and look up at its bank of lights in the darkness. We can walk toward the red glow that spells out the word EMERGENCY above a lighted arrow, a direction only last month I walked myself. And as we move through that space, I'll ask you how it is that on the sixth floor cancer ward women wake through Demerol and beg to live, and three flights up in the psychiatric ward they sink into Xanax and beg to die. Are there two hells for women, each distinct?

God, what am I doing? I sound like the women in the audience of my own poetry readings. The ones who think they know me, who slip me notes and telephone numbers, who afterward have to tell me about their own diagnoses and breakdowns and ask what they should do. The benefit reading for the women's crisis center was the worst. How I just wanted to scream, "Get away, it's just poetry, how do you know what I say is about me? I have a Ph.D. and a good prognosis. I don't live there anymore." Don't you hate reverence, Audre?

All that worship of blood, and moon, and soil?

In truth, I said nothing. I said none of this as I swam the current of awkwardness toward her. I sat on the shoreline, wild and half-drowned, brimming with confession, saying nothing. I remember she held my hand between both of hers. She asked me, "Have I given you everything you need from me tonight?" And still disbelieving, I shook my head. Finally I said, "Yes, oh, yes, yes, yes." And she answered, "Your mouth is saying yes, but your head is saying no. What do you mean?"

Notes:

1. "I memorized your words": The quote by Audre Lorde is from *The Cancer Journals* (San Francisco: Spinsters/Aunt Lute, 1980) p.75. Lorde died of breast cancer in 1992.

2. The Huron River runs by the University of Michigan Hospital in Ann Arbor.

# The Politics of Cancer

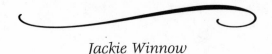

*Jackie Winnow*

EVERYTHING ABOUT CANCER IS POLITICAL, and that's the way we have to look at it. As lesbians and feminists, we need to be making connections and analyzing what the media presents to us, what the media tells us, about cancer and how then we react to it. And we have to know what the realities in our lives are, rather than what the media or the American Cancer Society tells us about what the realities of our lives are once we get cancer. That's the only way we can change things.

All of these centers [feminist and lesbian cancer projects], every one of these centers, is political. The fact that we as feminists, the fact that we as lesbians, have created these centers as a consumer-feminist movement is so political. Somebody who was putting together a politics of cancer anthology once asked me why she should include the Mautner Project because it was direct services to lesbians. I said, "If you don't understand why a direct service agency to lesbians is political, you don't really understand anything—you've just put together the anthology."

I think it's really important for us to look at the fact that cancer is being controlled from the top to the bottom. It's been controlled by professionals, by the American Cancer Society, by the petroleum companies, by the chemical companies, by the Rockefellers. The fact that we have taken control, once again, as feminists and lesbians, is a really political act and has been very threatening to the cancer establishment, and there is a tremendous cancer establishment in this country that profits from it.

I'd like to give you a little bit of a personal background on me before I go on, so you can get a small understanding of where I'm coming from. I'm making my part of this as brief as I can. I usually talk endlessly. Maybe it has something to do with cancer. Anyway, in 1985 I was diagnosed with breast cancer, in Oakland, California. In the period of a weekend between my biopsy and my diagnosis, my lover Teya and I realized that we had to become cancer experts. So we did become cancer experts over the weekend. The day I got my diagnosis of breast cancer, I had been in a meeting. I was the coordinator of Lesbian/Gay and AIDS Unit of the San Francisco Human Rights Commission. We just had spent five or six hours at a meeting on AIDS, and all I was thinking about in this meeting was "my biopsy results, my biopsy results." When my surgeon called me at ten o'clock that night, I knew it was bad news. I had negative nodes, which was supposed to be a good diagnosis. I had a lumpectomy followed by radiation, and what happened to me in the reality of the situation was there was no place to go to empower myself. There was no central information source to empower myself to become an informed consumer for my own health care. And that was stunning to me.

We had feminist health centers, if I had a yeast infection, and we had AIDS centers, if I had AIDS, but we had nothing established for ourselves as far as cancer was concerned. So it was catch as catch can. Another woman, named Carla Dalton, and myself became known as "the cancer mavens." And everybody just started calling us all the time. We decided that really what we needed to do was create a center [the Women's Cancer Resource Center in Berkeley]. The center was to be a central resource center, so that people could come and get support and information, and come and agitate about cancer. But the basic underlying point of the center is empowerment: so that women become empowered to make the decisions they need to make to live the lives that they need to live. . . . We started in late 1986 planning it. Before we knew it, we had to have a support group, because the idea of it became so—there was such a need. It was unbelievable. It all blossomed before we could really do our proper planning.

The American Cancer Society let us use their kitchen. We started our support groups, and they sent people to us. That's how our support group was started, so that as we were organizing we kept something going to meet people's needs. But people kept on thinking—because we got all this media attention too—that there was this big center, and really it was just part of the study in my house. The phone was in there, and that's how we started. We needed to start before we started, so it all just became this big circle.

In 1988 I was diagnosed with metastatic breast cancer to my lungs and bones, and that's why it's hard to me to talk loud, because of the cancer in my lungs, and it's hard for me to sit, because of the cancer in my bones. But in taking care of my own business and becoming weaker than I had been, the leadership of the center is falling apart, so Susan Liroff, who is now director, stepped in there and took it off, and it's been really wonderful. We have our own place. It's as environmentally safe as we can get it, and we have a library. We have information referral. We have many different kinds of support groups. We have an educational program. We have a speaker's bureau, and we just have a lot of different kinds of activities. We wish we could have more, but there's just so much we can do at a time. We're just moving along in that direction.

Now, with the history of all that behind us, I think it's so exciting to see what's happening to women's programs, to see that we have created this movement, that there are now centers, that there are political action groups that are agitating on our behalf. It's very exciting that people are seeing cancer as a political issue in a society that tries to keep cancer as a personal issue. People get cancer, and it's this personal issue, and you take care of it yourself. Louis Sullivan, U.S. Secretary of Health, came out with a 600-page report about how Americans can take care of their own health care, and it was basically a 600-page report about pulling yourself up by your own bootstraps. There was no mention of national health care; there was no mention of what the corporations could do to clean up the environment or change their behavior as far as cancer was concerned. I think that we have incorporated very much the idea of individual responsibility for cancer, and we in the feminist community have done the same thing because we live in this world. It is not incidental that Louis Sullivan talks about cancer in a private way or health care in a private way. When you have Louise Hay who talks about cancer as being a personal, emotional problem, you've got Bernie Seigel asking you why you need to have it, and you've got a lot of psychobabble about why people have cancer, because there is no cure for cancer and they don't really know the causes of cancer. So here it is: people have their personal problems and that's why they have cancer, rather than the fact that there are biological and molecular things going on in the body that are being promoted by a noxious world.

We see it in our own community: if I have positive thinking, I won't get cancer; if I run, I won't get cancer; if I eat properly, I won't get cancer. So what did you do to get cancer?

We're going to have to look at that. There's this whole thing that we create our own reality, so if you sit and you visualize, you can visualize away your cancer and if you don't do it, then there's something wrong with you. You've got fear. People get cancer because they fear love, and if you didn't fear love, then you wouldn't have cancer. Love has nothing to do with it. Give me a break. And then we've got karma. Karma comes back again. This is big stuff, you know. People make a lot of money out of it. We incorporate it into ourselves too. And when you hold the individuals accountable for this disease, then the culprits go scott-free.

We've got an incredible epidemic happening in our country, and I'm going to give you some of those statistics, so that you get a handle on how incredible this epidemic really is. One in three Americans now gets cancer in their lifetime. In 1950, it was one in ten. That's an incredible jump in a very short period of time. So when we talk about people living longer, etc., etc., we're talking in 1950 it was one in ten and now it's one in three. There are five million people in the United States who have cancer. One million people are going to be diagnosed with this disease this year, and half a million people are going to die. Half a million people. And if we say that a million people are going to get cancer this year, and we're ten percent of the population, then we're talking about 100,000 lesbians being diagnosed with cancer this year. One hundred years ago, cancer caused less than three percent of the deaths in the United States. Today it kills one in four men. When I was diagnosed with breast cancer in 1985, one in eleven women got breast cancer, and now it's one in nine. [1]

The rate for breast cancer for women between the ages 30 and 35 has tripled since 1977 and quadrupled for women between the ages of 35 and 39. That's amazing. It was once considered an "old lady's" disease. It is no longer considered an old lady's disease. 175,000 women will get breast cancer this year, and 45,000 will die from this disease. The thing that's really startling about this is that we have a lot of positive stuff coming out from the American Cancer Society about all that's been done for cancer. And breast cancer, the statistics for breast cancer have not changed since 1930: it's been the same amount of women dying from breast cancer now as they did in 1930. [2] They may live longer, but they die at the same rate. So nothing has really changed.

When they talk about prevention, they are talking about early detection. If you find a lump in a mammogram, you already have cancer. You haven't prevented a damn thing. So you have to understand, they haven't come up with anything to prevent cancer, only things that detect it earlier, and then they pass it off as prevention.

We can do things to change, individually. We can stop smoking. We can change our diets. We can exercise. We can do some of those things to take care of ourselves. But we can't think of ourselves as living in a vacuum, in that we are responsible for our health, because we cannot be ultimately responsible for our health. We don't control everything in our environment. We know that as lesbians we don't control the society.

Prevention would be the proliferation of these kinds of centers in the system that change the system, that change the structure of the system. There should be national health care in this society. We don't have national health care. People are not getting health care. Black women are being diagnosed with cancer at a much greater rate than white women and . . . are much more likely to die from it.

The Women's Health Trial was being developed for eight years. It had to do with breast cancer and diet and the fact that a low-fat diet might affect cancer. Feminists tried to put the Women's Health Trial through three different times, and on three different occasions they were told it was too difficult for the government researchers to carry it through, that women would not change their diets, and that it was too difficult to do a diet where women had to change their diet, because you couldn't trust them. It wasn't like giving them a pill. Of course, they've done a *lot* of studies on heart disease and diet, and I guess men can change their diets and they don't have to give them a pill and they can trust them. But they would not put the money into this, to see what would happen with women. At the same time, women's groups began lobbying the NCI (the National Cancer Institute) and the National Institutes of Health, and they promised to give us more money and they promised to fund a study, and the third time they denied the study. And one of the reasons they said they denied the study was because they wouldn't be able to reach all socioeconomic groups because you couldn't trust Black women to eat a low-fat diet. That was one of the reasons that they gave.

But under some stress from people like us, because we are organizing, because we have people like Pat Schroeder in office, and we have Olympia Snow and we have Barbara Milkulski, they have formed a women's congressional committee and have proposed the Women's Health Equity Act, which is twelve separate bills dealing with women's health issues. It was discovered that hardly any, *any* medical trials were being done on women at all. Although we're 52 percent of the population, the National Cancer Institute was spending 13 percent of its budget on women. We're 52 percent of the population. They've now doubled it to 26 percent, but it's still only 26 percent.

It's really important for us to look at that and keep on pushing this feminist agenda in the Congress, because it has gotten somewhere and we need to keep on doing it. What I'm very concerned about right now is that there's a new women's cancer national organization being put together, but it's being put together to deal with breast cancer and breast cancer issues. I think at this point in our organizing, because we are starting these organizations, we need to build a national agenda to deal with women and cancer. Not just breast cancer, because we don't only get breast cancer and women are not just defined by their tits, or their lack thereof. It's very important for us to see and not exclude women who have all different kinds of cancer and to make sure that everybody knows that we do get other kinds of cancer besides breast cancer, including lung cancer at increasing rates, as the cigarette companies are targeting women in their ads to smoke.

We talk about prevention and we have a government that keeps on throwing out that we shouldn't be smoking, but they support the tobacco industry. So where are our tax dollars going?

We have to look very closely when we're talking about prevention and when we're organizing. At the petrochemical companies, we have to see what happened in 1950 that is so different from now. What happened in 1950 is that we had the beginning of the petrochemical companies. We had radiated Nagasaki and Hiroshima, and we had underground and overground testing everywhere of radiation in this country, in the deserts. We had chemical companies starting to make chemicals; we had chemical dumping. We had toxic waste dumps, and they've found that toxic waste dumps are more likely to happen in neighborhoods where poor people and people of color live. We have no ozone layer—I mean we have an ozone layer, but we're having holes there.

We have a food chain that has become mass-produced. Before 1950, we didn't have a mass-produced food chain, and we have that now. The animals are fed massive antibiotics and toxins, and they live in incredibly terrible conditions. And they're bred simply for mass-production rather than for any nutritional value. And then you've got your vegetables that are sprayed with pesticides everywhere; you've got your farmworkers who are dying in the fields because they're being sprayed by the pesticides; and somehow, even though the farmworkers are dying of the pesticide spraying, we're not supposed to question that they are in fact picking the food that has those pesticides and we're eating it. And then we have all this stuff that's gone into the water.

So what we're talking about is changing the system that works for profits rather than people. That is the point. This society doesn't care whether we die. We are the throwaways, because we don't own chemical companies, and even if we did there are other major stockholders, and people are making profit. It's the profit-making system of this country that brings us into wars and that makes us kill our own people here at home. We need national health care. We need an end to the sexist, demeaning attitude toward women and health care, and we need it throughout this whole society. Otherwise, it's not going to work when we try to change health care. We need to clean up the environment. We need to make connections to other movements for social change rather than to think that it's an individual solution. And we have to start our own self-help programs because we have to take back our own health care.

We have to support our own local service centers. We have to build some more. One of the things that is really telling to me is when I have done speeches and women have called me up who are disabled to say that there are no longer any attendants. There used to be a lot of lesbian attendants for them, and there no longer are as many lesbian attendants because they're working with men who have AIDS. And I'm not pitting us against men who have AIDS, because I think men who have AIDS need help and women with AIDS need help. What I am saying is that we also have to put our energies into women's health care. We don't have to take it out. We need to put it back in. We need to be there for them.

When we are dealing with fundraising, when we are working for lesbians, we have to make sure that we understand the cancer politics and cancer realities. That goes for all of us. We need to be changing billboards, so that the presence is brought home. Somebody changed a billboard in San Francisco for the movie *Marked for Death* to read "Marked for death. 1000 women a day marked for death by the NCI." It was very effective immediately.

How can you question the National Cancer Institute? I heard a figure given from the stage last night that six percent less funding is given to cancer research now than it was ten years ago. And we have to have research that's valuable research rather than research that just goes for a bullet type of cure. We have to have research that deals with the realities of people's lives. We have to elect women to office, and we have to move for legislation, and we really have to be marching in the streets. I think we really have to understand how urgent this is, because women are getting cancer, women are dying from cancer at ever-increasing rates, and our lives depend on what we do in this room today.

Notes:
1. This was April 1991. As of November 1992, it was one in eight.
2. Winnow was referring to the fact that the number of women dying has increased dramatically; the percentage of women dying compared to the number of women being diagnosed has remained the same.

This article is a transcription of a talk given by Jackie Winnow at the first meeting of representatives of the first four grassroots women's/feminist/lesbian community cancer projects (in Oakland, Boston, Washington, D.C., and Chicago) at the National Lesbian Conference in Atlanta, Georgia, in April 1991.

# Closure

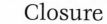

*Teya Schaffer*

*i*

It is not like drowning any more:
your life no longer a silent film
flickering before my eyes.
No, now you are wrapped like a holy text
over arm and forehead, enscrolled
on the doorposts of my house,
a commandment of remembrance.

*ii*

I am not done.
I am not finished missing you.
How could memory forget its creator?
the ungiven future would have found us
seeking still the persuasive truths
which show the beloved her beauty;
how could memory forget its purpose?

First I loved you
true and well.
You loved me like a tree:
canopy and root.
In those days I could speak your name
in all the public places.
When you were dying
your name became a wreath
on my brow, marking me
as more than I was;
people took your name from my lips
and poured it burning into my ears.
You were a burning crown
and now are ash:
a future bereft of prediction
a silence caught in the teeth.

your name was Jackie
when you mocked my vanities
my heart was comforted
when you nested your fears in my heart
my courage was sufficient
when you broke my heart with refusal
I still was whole
when my failings tripped your strength
your love was not diminished
what if death is unceasing
there are other things
which last as long

# The New Year

*Teya Schaffer*

*i*

Conveniently our street ends in the cemetery where we
used to take the baby in his stroller, bicyclists and joggers
more common than mourners. We make an appointment,
"pre-need." Learn prices and locales. The number of
people allowed in each plot varies with terrain and
container, casket or urn. Stones must lie flat. We are
already out of our bodies just being there.

At least the quarrel is behind us, of where to rest in
perpetual care. Generic ground spreads near the entrance.
The old Jewish section is lovely but filled; the new one,
treeless as a subdivision, is a long mile uphill. She refuses to
be buried "in a ghetto." I won't lie "among strangers."
First going gets first dibs; I give way and see her desire:
that there be passersby to read her name.

She prepares for her death with a to-do list, a lined yellow
pad at the ready. We research mortuaries because it's our
habit to know, to care, our questions a parody of the
search for health. Who will touch her body? How long can
it stay at home? We want refrigeration, not embalming. I
go without her to the showroom. "Not 'cheap,'" a wincing
salesperson corrects me, "'inexpensive.'" Either way I
choose her box; consult at home, "lined or not?" At Albert
Brown's I'm warned away from washing her myself—
death's not pretty, the consultant says. So I go with Chapel
of the Chimes. How do I go on, walking down the street,
buying the child his dinner? From her bed she hands me
the yellow tablet: a penciled rectangle, name, dates,
beloved.

The hidden businesses are revealed. Goodbye to the local
pharmacy and its line of caregivers buying Tylenol with
codeine and Ensure. On to the farther one, smaller and
darker, which sells morphine. In come the supplies, the rail
for the toilet, the i.v. pole and its bags of saline. Out goes
our mattress in the arms of a stranger returning with a cot
and a hospital bed. We sit in the midst, with a hospice
nurse disappointed by our talk of nausea when she'd hoped
for our souls. In the quieter hours we keep to two rooms,
quietly dying, quietly stitching a rose.

Her death reads like a book, the labored and infrequent
breaths pages from a year of study; friends and family pose
in quiet vignettes. The child comes to sit in my lap, his
hands colder than hers; then he leaves with an uncle. The
cats follow their needs, one curls by her face, the other on

a high shelf ready to thump down with her last breath.
Outside the window and two floors below, a band is
playing for some undeclared holiday, a merchants'
celebration. In between her rattling sounds, rise
unmistakable bars of "When the Saints Come Marching
In." The telephone rings, someone wants to know if she's
still here. The cat comes down.

*v*

I ask for privacy. I close the door; pull back the blanket;
remove the catheter. Join you. The press of my body
releases a final sigh from yours. My fingers discover the
you without you, greeting and leaving your toes and the
spaces between your toes, right foot and left, ankle and
shin, the manner of your walk, knee and thigh, the
memory of fat, hip and buttocks, my palm mating the
curve of pubic bone hello goodbye the skin of your
abdomen, the shadows beneath your breasts, your breasts
and the breast which betrayed us hello goodbye scars   the
hollow of your collarbone   the sparse hairs beneath your
arm   the inside of your elbow   the stilled veins   the narrow
wrist   the fit of our hands   the turn of my face into your
neck. This is the moment we have waited for; I won't
leave it for years.

*vi*

Wash cloths, basin. Someone asks "shampoo?" three say
"no need." Her dying was clean, her body not impure,
still we understand: before going into the dirt she must
be touched by water. Soft terry barely damp, a murmur
of direction as we lift and lower; mother, sister, friend,
spouse, tenderly, thoroughly, smoothing our way over her
going. Her eyes half-open, as if this is something she would
like to see.

*Teya Schaffer*

## vii

I cross the threshold, carrying her like a bird in my mouth;
recognize the shapes of people as I move towards an empty
room. Marvelous the stillness of their language, the
sympathy in their distance, as if they too feel the concussed
air rippling between us. A way is being made for the
widow, on its quiet I place my feet.

## viii

There are no Sunday gravediggers. Consternation and
phone calls. Jews bury their dead on the following day
unless that day is forbidden for mourning. Her friends get
busy: she was a person of connections, maybe there are
strings to pull. Her sister asks if the photographs, brought
too late for viewing, can be buried with her. A friend offers
stones. They are coming for her body. We pull crayon
drawings off the refrigerator, a ribbon rose from the
dresser—don't be lonely, don't forget us, here's something
for the journey we don't believe you take.

I flee when the doorbell rings, return, after her body's
gone, with new wisdom: she is dead, she can wait until
Monday. Monday is the New Year, a forbidden day, but I
don't care. We never cared for rituals we couldn't use.

## ix

All I am asked to do is breathe. Her mother offers gin. Her
sister a sleeping pill. They are good gifts. In the morning
they bring me tea and toast. We blame our exhaustion on
the visitors and look forward to their return. It is right and
good, this ingathering of mourners to verify a loss, their
offerings of food. I remove the flower someone has placed
on her pillow, try not to wince when someone sits on
her bed.

*x*

Tomorrow we go to the cemetery. Tonight it is erev Rosh Hashanah. I prepare apples and honey, share with my son the sweetness of life. My tongue cradles the bird in my mouth, tells her the new year will never come.

# IN OUR OWN HANDS: A Brief History
## of the Lesbian Cancer Movement

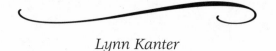

*Lynn Kanter*

IN 1929 A VOLUNTEER ARMY OF WOMEN set out to conquer cancer. They were recruited by the American Society to Control Cancer, and their mission was to spread its gospel: Put yourself and your family under a doctor's supervision immediately.[1] The Society had been founded in 1913 by a life insurance statistician who mobilized doctors and policymakers to increase the public's understanding of cancer. The disease could be controlled, the Society believed, by excising it decisively and unconditionally at the first sign of a tumor. And who better to convince women of the importance of taking swift action than other women? After all, women were responsible not only for themselves but for the health of their entire families. So the battalions of women volunteers spread the word, distributing some 668,000 copies of a pamphlet called "What Every Woman Should Know about Cancer." They passed out this vast number of pamphlets one at a time, hand to hand, at women's clubs and cocktail parties and family gatherings, at schools and shops and anywhere women were likely to meet other women in the white, affluent enclaves that constituted the known world as defined by the Society.

By 1933 this army of volunteers had moved from the metaphorical to the material, as more than one hundred thousand women paid one dollar each to join the Society's newly established Women's Field Army. Each soldier dedicated herself to encouraging women to get checkups, to recognize the symptoms of cancer and to seek immediate treatment if they spotted the warning signs. The Women's Field Army also mounted public relations campaigns, conducted public education programs and helped to establish the nation's earliest cancer prevention clinics. The volunteers could not help noticing that the lifesaving measures they advocated so fervently were unavailable to poor women. Unlike the male medical establishment at whose behest they were working, many members of the Women's Field Army took action to ameliorate this injustice, financing cancer treatment for low-income women. In doing so, the dedicated volunteers provoked the hostility of physicians who suspected them of practicing socialism.

The Women's Field Army operated for approximately ten years, mobilizing some three hundred thousand women in thirty-nine states. Never intended to be radical, the organization enlisted for the most part white, heterosexual, married, middle-class women to advance the cancer agenda of the medical fraternity. But in its galvanizing of women volunteers, its smashing of the taboos against speaking aloud the word "cancer," its demonstration of the power women possess to change and save each other's lives, this army of women broke the path for the next generation of cancer activists. In 1945 the American Society to Control Cancer evolved into the American Cancer Society. Within three years the organization had taken over what remained of the dwindling activities of the Women's Field Army.

During World War II government and industry had successfully used the power of advertising to persuade middle-class women to prove their patriotism by working in factories and other outposts of the war effort. When the war ended, this propaganda machine just as forcefully urged women to hand over their jobs to the returning veterans and retire to their preordained place in the kitchen and nursery. Activist Betty Friedan challenged that destiny in her 1963 manifesto, *The Feminine Mystique*. The book helped to spark a women's liberation movement that fundamentally transformed women's understanding of their roles, their options and their power in society.

One of the most contested issues was the question of who "owned" women's bodies. Far from a theoretical concern, this issue gave rise to fierce struggles over reproductive rights and to the then novel idea that rape and domestic violence were serious crimes.

The contest for the control of women's bodies also led to the radical realization that women's health itself was a political issue, shaped by fundamental conflicts over access to information, to health care, to treatment options and to that rarest of all medical commodities—respect for women as patients, as practitioners and as decision-makers. As this second wave of feminism swept across the nation during the sixties and early seventies, it inspired American women to view their own health in a new, and angrier, light. In growing numbers they took action to demystify medicine, to provide affordable health services, to end the male monopoly on the practice of medicine and to force medical institutions to take women's illnesses seriously and to stop treating normal life processes (pregnancy and menopause, for example) as illnesses.

In 1970 the Boston Women's Health Book Collective published Our Bodies, Ourselves, one of the first works to offer a comprehensive look at diverse aspects of women's health from an explicitly feminist point of view. Within six years the book had sold more than a million copies.[2] A survey conducted by the New York–based HealthRight collective in 1973 identified more than a thousand feminist health projects that were active nationwide.[3] Just a glance at some of the names of those projects provides a sense of how rich and widespread the level of activity was: the Somerville Women's Health Project in Massachusetts; the Fremont Women's Clinic in Seattle; the Feminist Women's Health Centers in Los Angeles and a dozen other sites; the Women's Information Service in Pueblo, Colorado; the Women's Rap Program in Tampa, Florida; and the Elizabeth Blackwell Brigade in Bellingham, Washington.

The year 1974 saw two events that would mark the dawn of the movement to fight breast cancer. First Lady Betty Ford broke the tradition of secrecy by going public with her diagnosis of breast cancer. Suddenly the words "breast cancer"—until recently discussed only in whispers or euphemisms—rang out from television screens and front pages throughout the land. But the most influential event of 1974 went almost unheralded. Rose Kushner was a science writer for the Washington Post who, like Ford, had recently been diagnosed with breast cancer. Kushner launched a pioneering campaign to transform the way Americans approached the disease and those who struggled with it. She published persuasive articles denouncing the fact that doctors told their patients so little about breast cancer that the women were unable to make informed decisions about treatment options. The information was available, Kushner wrote, but "as inaccessible to most women as the files of the CIA and the FBI."[4]

What was worse, doctors routinely made the most critical decision—to pursue the most radical surgical approach, a mastectomy, which Kushner called "amputating a woman's breast"—without consulting the patient, before she had even regained consciousness after her surgical biopsy. Kushner was among the first and most vociferous advocates of a two-step process: a surgical biopsy followed by a candid discussion with the woman about her treatment options. "Most physicians will say that a woman is committing suicide if she waits, but this is a myth," she declared. "Women can safely wait as long as two weeks after a biopsy to get opinions" from other physicians.[5] In 1975 Kushner published her ground-breaking book, *Breast Cancer: A Personal History and an Investigative Report*, which challenged for the first time the medical establishment's unexamined, illogical and often cruel treatment of women with breast cancer.

That same year, the National Women's Health Network was founded and held its first national conference, attracting thirteen hundred women. Also in 1975 women from a variety of organizations lobbied in Washington, D.C., to protest the continued use of diethylstilbestrol (DES), an artificial estrogen that was widely prescribed to pregnant women although it was known to cause a rare and often fatal gynecological cancer in the daughters and testicular cancer in the sons of women who took the drug.

Lesbians led this vital, varied and energetic women's health movement. They were in the forefront of the feminist struggles for reproductive rights, the founders of the grassroots organizations, the workers in clinics, the fighters for resources and policies. Later AIDS created a new arena in which lesbians played a critical role as organizers and as caregivers. In the late 1970s and early 1980s health clinics for lesbians began to emerge, such as the Lyon-Martin Women's Health Clinic in San Francisco. In 1981 the Gay and Lesbian Medical Association, then called the American Association of Physicians for Human Rights, was founded by doctors dedicated to combating homophobia in the medical profession and promoting quality health care for all. But for the most part, lesbians were taking care of everyone else first and themselves last—or not at all.

A lesbian, a feminist and a prominent AIDS activist, Jackie Winnow was a perfect example. When she was diagnosed with cancer in 1985 she found no source of assistance in the San Francisco Bay Area, where she and others had worked so hard to establish systems of support for HIV-positive people. In 1986 she rallied a small group of cancer survivors and created the Women's Cancer Resource Center in Berkeley, California—the nation's first feminist cancer project. For the first two years of the center's existence, twenty volunteers took turns returning messages left on an answering machine in a volunteer's home. The calls were mostly from women who had recently been diagnosed with cancer and wanted information and support. As word of mouth grew about this new resource, so did the volunteer pool, and the fledgling organization developed into a strong presence in the community and in national cancer advocacy circles. Today the center serves all women with cancer, and the open leadership and involvement of lesbians has contributed immensely to the organization's vibrancy. The center has a staff of four and more than 120 volunteers "dedicated to the radical notion that women are entitled to information, services, support and understanding," as the organization's Web site proclaims.[6]

Throughout the 1980s many women found themselves radicalized and politicized by cancer. For example, women in Long Island discovered that their breast cancer rates were 10 to 20 percent higher than those of women throughout the rest of New York State.[7] They were relieved to hear that the state was conducting a major study to ascertain the reason for this alarmingly high incidence. When journalist Joan Swirsky learned that the study wasn't even examining the possible role of drinking water or toxic dumpsites, she used her newspaper column to demand changes in the study design.[8] Thanks to the activism of Swirsky and other women, the study was twice redesigned. But when the research was completed after five years, the results absolved environmental factors from all responsibility and instead concluded that affluence was the primary contributing factor to the high breast cancer rate.

Out of the fury that followed these findings grew One in Nine, a breast cancer advocacy group comprised of survivors and supporters. When the Centers for Disease Control and Prevention (CDC) refused to recommend a new study, "women took matters into their own hands," ecologist and cancer-survivor Sandra Steingraber wrote in her 1997 book *Living Downstream: An Ecologist Looks at Cancer and the Environment.*[9] "Some [women] began creating their own maps" of cancer clusters, Steingraber reported. "In the fall of 1993, a group of activists hosted their own scientific conference, the first in the nation to bring together scientists and women with cancer to design a program of study." Finally, in 1994, the New York State Department of Health produced a study that linked cancer risk with residence near chemical plants.

The history of the lesbian and feminist cancer movement is illuminated by inspiring books and articles that pointed out a new path for activists and reshaped the way people thought about cancer. Writer-activist Audre Lorde's 1980 book, *The Cancer Journals*, was such a revelation. Jackie Winnow's article "Lesbians Evolving Health Care," first published in *Out/Look* in 1989, was another. Equally influential was "Cancer as a Feminist Issue," written by activist-journalist Susan Shapiro and published in 1989 in the Boston-based feminist journal *Sojourner*. In that article Shapiro applied a scathing feminist analysis to women's experience of breast cancer, including her own. She invited women to gather to discuss the issue, and twenty-five women responded. From that meeting emerged the Women's Community Cancer Project (WCCP), based in Cambridge, Massachusetts. The WCCP's mission is to change "the current social, medical and political approaches to cancer, particularly as they affect women."[10] Comprised of lesbian, straight and bisexual women whose lives have been affected by cancer, this grassroots volunteer organization is known especially for its well-researched fact sheets on cancer and related health issues. Many of the political approaches Shapiro advocated have been adopted by cancer advocacy groups across the country. But sadly she did not live to see the benefits: Shapiro died of breast cancer at age thirty-eight, only four months after the first meeting of the organization she cofounded.

Lawyer Mary-Helen Mautner also wrote a document that, despite never being published, triggered a movement. Mautner was a forty-four-year-old mother and lesbian feminist activist who had been a member of the radical Furies collective, among many other political involvements. One day in the summer of 1989, as she lay immobile while a bone scan measured her spreading breast cancer, Mautner reflected on how lucky she was. She thought about her dedicated partner in life and in activism, Susan Hester. She thought about the dozens of friends who had helped them take care of their young daughter and handle daily chores while she and Hester confronted the immense burden of catastrophic illness. And she thought about the lesbians who didn't have such resources, who had to face alone the practical and emotional—and political—ordeals of cancer.

Mautner imagined an organization that would provide assistance and support to lesbians with cancer and their families in the Washington, D.C., area. She jotted down her ideas in a note that was both powerful for the vision and thoroughness it reflected and poignant for what it lacked—any mention of a role for herself in organizing the initiative. Three weeks later she died. In early 1990, Hester and other Washington-area activists founded the Mary-Helen Mautner Project for Lesbians with Cancer—the first grassroots cancer project in the nation dedicated to serving the lesbian community. During its first year of existence, the growing cadre of Mautner Project volunteers found themselves immensely busy. They launched a weekly support group for lesbians with cancer, drove women to medical treatments, assisted women in applying for entitlement programs, established a blood-donor registry and coordinated blood donations. Volunteers spoke at lesbian and gay events, presented workshops at national gatherings and participated in mainstream professional conferences, where lesbian issues had rarely if ever been raised.

Volunteers soon took on another activity that would mark the Mautner Project's place in the lesbian cancer movement. They advised and encouraged lesbians in Chicago who were working to establish their own cancer group, the Chicago Lesbian Community Cancer Project, founded in October 1990. The following year, the Mautner Project assisted women in Philadelphia in organizing the Lesbian Cancer Network.

By 1991 the women of the Mautner Project realized that they had to do more. It was not enough to care for the sick and comfort the survivors, not enough to educate and inform. Although the project served lesbians with all kinds of cancer, breast cancer seemed to be cutting a horrifying swath through the community, not only in Washington, D.C., but nationwide. Mary-Helen Mautner, Jackie Winnow, the activist-writers Audre Lorde, Pat Parker and Barbara Rosenblum—breast cancer had taken them all. It was time to fight back, time to focus public attention and political energy on the seemingly unnoticed public health crisis of breast cancer. It was time to organize.

The Mautner Project had gained a strong supporter in Dr. Susan M. Love, author of the 1990 *Dr. Susan Love's Breast Book,* a nationally known breast cancer expert. Love believed that "the cure for breast cancer is political action."[11] In 1991 she flew to Washington to headline the project's first educational event. During that visit Love and several Mautner Project volunteers talked intently about the breast cancer movement, comparing its placid pace with the fire of the AIDS movement. They determined that breast cancer needed its own national political movement to press for progress in finding a cure. Several weeks later, Love and Hester met with Amy Langer of the National Alliance of Breast Cancer Organizations to brainstorm about which cancer organizations could be called together to trigger such a campaign. Sparked by two lesbians schooled in activism, the meetings that followed resulted in the creation of the National Breast Cancer Coalition in 1994.

The first national advocacy effort to address breast cancer, the coalition was also the first nationwide health advocacy group to have a lesbian organization—the Mautner Project for Lesbians with Cancer—on its board of directors. Over the past few years the coalition has taken the lead in training and organizing women across the country to demand expanded federal funding for breast cancer research. Their activism played an important role in achieving an increase in research funds from $90 million a year when the coalition began to $660 million in 1999.[12]

In 1994 the Mautner Project established an unprecedented partnership with the Avon Breast Cancer Awareness Crusade, which for the first time recognized lesbians as an under-served population and funded the project's efforts to expand breast cancer education and screening within the lesbian community. That same year the Mautner Project helped organize the first briefing ever given to the CDC on lesbians and cancer. In that historic meeting, lesbian health advocates from across the country made the case that lesbians are medically under-served, facing discrimination and misinformation from health care providers. Through ongoing advocacy, the Mautner Project and other groups convinced the CDC to identify lesbians as a targeted population that requires special outreach to increase their access to health care and cancer screening. Today the project is implementing a million-dollar grant from the CDC to design a national training program to increase the "cultural competency" of health care providers, so they can better serve lesbians and their families.

From these pioneering beginnings—the independent actions of lesbians and feminists facing cancer in communities across the country—has grown a powerful and vibrant movement. Today lesbian cancer projects are active in Atlanta, Chicago, Denver, Jacksonville (Florida), Narragansett (Rhode Island), Portland (Oregon), Seattle and elsewhere. In January 2000 a new lesbian cancer organization, Wendy's Hope, opened in Los Angeles. Women's cancer projects, many of which operate with the energy of lesbian leadership and volunteers, and lesbian health programs that include cancer care components are at work in more than a dozen other cities. The lesbian cancer movement has been limited by the dearth of data about cancer in the lesbian community. The first large-scale study of lesbian health issues, the National Lesbian Health Care Survey, provided invaluable information but was not designed to address cancer risk or incidence. Authored by Dr. Caitlin Ryan and published by the National Gay and Lesbian Health Foundation in 1987, this ground-breaking survey was one of the few data sources available when Dr. Suzanne Haynes conducted her research on breast cancer. An epidemiologist at the National Cancer Institute, Haynes created shockwaves in 1993 when she estimated that lesbians might have a risk of developing breast cancer that is two to three times greater than the risk faced by heterosexual women. Her bold and controversial claim was widely misquoted as a "one in three risk."

Today scientists are for the first time amassing reliable research data that can serve as the basis for informed decision-making in both medical and the policy arenas. This is largely thanks to the dogged advocacy of lesbian cancer groups and the determination of researchers such as Haynes, Ryan, Dr. Judy Bradford, Dr. Stephanie Roberts, Dr. Deb Bowen and many others. The federally funded Women's Health Initiative—one of the largest research projects ever attempted—has recruited lesbian participants and asks all participants questions about sexual behavior that will enable researchers to compare risk factors for lesbians with other population groups.[13] These questions would not have been included without intense grassroots pressure on the National Institutes of Health from lesbian health activists around the country, notably Dr. Kate O'Hanlan and health policy expert Marj Plumb, former public policy director of the Gay and Lesbian Medical Association. The Lyon-Martin Women's Health Services facility in San Francisco is at work on a three-year study comparing the risk of breast cancer for lesbians and heterosexual women in California. Harvard's long-term study of women nurses now includes questions about sexual identity and behavior, thanks to more than a year of advocacy by lesbian health activists.[14]

The extent of the contributions of closeted lesbians who fought to eradicate cancer, from the soldiers of the Women's Field Army to the volunteers working in community cancer projects today may never be known. But the achievements of lesbian cancer activists nationwide who created with their sweat and their courage the resources, the research and the respect for lesbian lives that has brought such sweeping progress in only a few years can certainly be celebrated. In many cases these efforts emerged out of suffering, the determined action of women living with cancer or of women supporting a loved one through the disease, and the commitment of women who had attended too many funerals. This impulse to turn anguish into action—the conviction that motivates grassroots advocacy and has moved so many women from private loss to public leadership—propels the lesbian cancer movement.

The movement is necessary because lesbians who are dealing with cancer should not have to negotiate a medical and social system that doesn't recognize their relationships or respect their differences. Lesbians deserve information and assistance that is specific to their needs and their way of life. In a 1994 survey of the doctors and doctors-in-training who belong to the Gay and Lesbian Medical Association, more than half of the respondents said they had observed their heterosexual colleagues provide substandard care or even deny care to lesbian and gay patients.[15] As Marj Plumb wrote, "I am the kind of lesbian who gets invited to meetings and asked to sit on committees because everyone knows I am a lesbian. But having to correct the heterosexual assumptions of my own medical providers makes me physically ill."[16]

"Doctors discriminate, researchers discriminate, insurers discriminate," Kathleen DeBold, the Mautner Project's director, told the *New York Times* on November 23, 1999.[17] "Cancer does not discriminate, and that's why these groups are so important."

Activist-psychotherapist Sandra Butler said it best when she wrote, "We are again shaping a movement and taking our lives into our own hands, for they are not safe anywhere else."[18]

Notes:
1. Much of this discussion of the historic role of volunteers in the cancer movement is drawn from Ellen Leopold, *A Darker Ribbon: Breast Cancer, Women, and their Doctors in the Twentieth Century* (Boston: Beacon, 1999).
2. Fruchter, Fatt, Booth and Leidel, "The Women's Health Movement: Where Are We Now?" In Claudia Dreifus ed., *Seizing Our Bodies: The Politics of Women's Health* (New York: Vintage, 1977), 272.
3. Ibid., xxiv.
4. Ibid., 190.
5. Ibid., 194.
6. See the Web site of the Women's Cancer Resource Center at www-geography.berkeley.edu:80/WCRC/2MAIN.HTM.
7. Sandra Steingraber, *Living Downstream: An Ecologist Looks at Cancer and the Environment* (Reading, Mass.: Addison-Wesley, 1997), 79.
8. Arditti and Schreiber, "Killing Us Quietly: Cancer, the Environment, and Women." In Midge Stocker, ed., *Confronting Cancer, Constructing Change: New Perspectives on Women and Cancer* (Chicago: Third Side Press, 1993), 252.
9. Steingraber, *Living Downstream*, 80.
10. See the Web site of the Women's Community Cancer Project at www.wccp-cancer-project.org.
11. Barbara Seaman, "Beyond the Halsted Radical." Available on *On the Issues* on-line at http:// www.echonyc.com/~on issues/f97books1.html.
12. See the Web site of the National Breast Cancer Coalition at www.natlbcc.org.
13. Bowen, Powers and Greenlee, "Lesbian Health Research." in Jocelyn White and Marissa C. Martínez, eds., *The Lesbian Health Book: Caring for Ourselves* (Seattle: Seal, 1997), 309.
14. Liz Galst, "Lesbians and Cancer Risk." *Mamm Magazine*, December/January 1999.
15. White and Martínez, *Lesbian Health Book*, p. 27.
16. Marj Plumb, M. N. A., "Butch Identity, Breast Reduction and the Chicago Cubs: The Effect of Gender and Class on Lesbian Access to Health Care." *Lesbian Health Book*, 43.
17. Kathleen DeBold, Science Section, *New York Times*, November 23, 1999.
18. Sandra Butler, in *Confronting Cancer, Constructing Change*, xxi.

# not// a story

*Ruthann Robson*

O.K. O.K. YOU'VE HEARD THIS BEFORE. Maybe you don't know the precise details, but you know the major themes and events. You know diagnosis, fear, chemotherapy, confusion, surgery, despair, radiation, hope and the search for alternative therapies. Maybe you don't want to know more. Maybe you don't care which chemical assaults which gene on the DNA double helix in hopes of halting its reproduction. Or the side effects of each antinausea drug administered to counteract the side effects of chemotherapy. Or how the technician presses a magic marker against the flesh to make the tattoo for radiation. Or what it feels like to have a surgeon admire his own work and call your incision "beautiful." I wouldn't want you to know these things. I don't wish this information on anyone. Well, maybe one or two people. Or maybe all writers. Novelists who need a convenient death for a minor character always seem to choose cancer. The character hasn't even been diagnosed yet and her hair is falling out in dramatic hunks. "Stupid asshole author," I want to scream, "it's the treatment that makes the hair fall out, not the disease." At least if I write about it, I'll be accurate. "Cancer isn't interesting." My editor says this. I don't tell her I have a rare and therefore maybe more intriguing form of cancer. Sarcoma. Sounds like a Greek isle, someplace I would like to live, somewhere between Sardinia and Lesbos, I imagine. Somewhere blue and healthy. I wanted to show my editor that I was still viable despite my newly fragile health, saying that perhaps I could craft art out of suffering. But my editor can be rather negative. I admit that I thought her comment was tactless, maybe even rude, and certainly insensitive. It's certainly not something I would ever say. But that may be the reason I have cancer and she doesn't. At least according to the pop psychologists. Keeping one's feelings to one's self is a sure signal to those wayward cancer cells that a body should be homesteaded. "Cancer can be depressing." My oncologist says this. She suggests a psychiatrist who could "prescribe something" in case I need help dealing with the diagnosis. Meaning the diagnosis that she has delivered in tones that make my editor sound like she's Miss Power-of-Positive-Thinking. It's as if my oncologist thinks if she says something that might be considered slightly optimistic and I die anyway, I'll sue her or something. She doesn't want to give what she calls "false hope."

If I had to have an oncologist, I wanted a woman. When I first met her, I felt reassured, comforted. Ambitious, she must be, and smart. Plus a lilt in her voice that could be seductive over a Bloody Mary or a Mimosa at brunch. But perhaps her line of work has made her grim. She can't even ask a question without putting me on a trajectory toward tragedy:

"Do you have any pain yet?"

"Are you still eating?"

"Have your feet started tingling?"

Am I just paranoid, or is she disappointed if the disease is not progressing on schedule?

She certainly isn't like the doctors who write those popular healing books, one of whom has the same editor as I do. These doctors are always positive and play symphonies during surgery to promote their patients' recovery. These doctors believe in miracles and the patients' abilities to defy all the statistics; they believe in anecdotes and individualism. They are writers of paperback nonfiction and readers of nineteenth-century novels. "Personal responsibility" is their mantra. Which is pretty close to blame, if you ask me.

What I am asked most, in the pop books and in the mountain of medical forms and in conversations with people I had been thinking were my friends is this: Did you smoke? I simply answer "no" and don't even explain that my particular kind of cancer isn't remotely respiratory. No one asks about high-tension wires, pesticides, working conditions, living near a toxic waste dump. I suppose that's not the kind of blame that's required. Not individual enough.

Then there's diet, although the medical profession is not as keen on this one. It is another disappointment that I'm a vegetarian. No McDonald's quarter pounders lurking in my bloodstream. Too much ice cream? Or maybe it was that cup of coffee in the morning. Didn't you have cheesecake in 1979? Though again, it doesn't seem to matter that my particular kind of cancer isn't digestive.

Sarcoma is a cancer of the connective tissues rather than the organs. Tissues like muscle, blood vessel, fat, bone, cartilage. Fewer than six thousand cases globally per year. No known cause. No known cure.

The psychologists don't care about cures. They speak of healing. You can be cured but unhealed, they say. Or you can be healed but dead. Do I get a choice, I want to ask?

The psychologists also don't care about causes like smoking or pollution or junk food, arguing that not everyone who smokes, or lives under high-tension wires, or eats a Big Mac with French fries every day gets cancer. Their variable is self-love. Let's talk about your parents. As if everyone with an un-loved inner child gets cancer?

Blame is a strategy of control. It separates the healthy from the sick and keeps us on our own sides. It tells the healthy that their fate is not their fate, but a product of their individual choices and completely within their own power, at least if they stop smoking, live in the right places, eat this week's correct foods and get enough psychotherapy. It makes the healthy feel safe.

Talk about false hope.

This is when I should mention how healthy I felt; how I went to the doctor for a rare checkup because I felt a strange lump that I would ordinarily have ignored except for the fact that I inadvertently mentioned it to my lover and she was insistent. This is when I should mention the exercise regimen I've followed for the past few years, the successes I was having, the way my entire life felt settled and right. This is when I should mention all that, make a list—

bookshelves, lover, tenure, child, novels, house, dog and cat, new clutch for the car—but if I do, my composition and my composure will decompose.

So, let me get back to my task. I guess I somehow believe that I can write my way out of this mess. The way I've written myself out of other messes, like heterosexuality for instance. I wrote and wrote and refused to read the novel of my life that had been handed to me when I was born: Its plotless plot was marriage to a man who worked on his car on Saturday afternoons and slapped me around on Saturday nights. I had affairs with women on the page long before I actually touched flesh. My still-childish handwriting assaulted the lined notebook paper with descriptions of breasts and legs, eyes and sweat, and of course, hair. I loved hair, including my own.

Especially my own.

It wandered to my waist and across my face. At night, I fanned it across my lovers' fantasy breasts. My fantasy lover looked a lot like the picture of Delilah in *The Children's Illustrated Book of Bible Stories*. She seemed to have long hair herself, but its provocative redness was twisted around her head so as not to obscure the curvaceous body barely covered by some leopard print outfit similar to what Wilma wore in *The Flintstones* cartoons. Which left me to imagine myself as Samson, who was certainly sexier than Fred Flintstone but a bit of a bore, going around killing Philistines with the jawbone of an ass. Still, he had that glorious long hair that was the source of his strength. Of course, the story ends badly—as love stories and Bible stories always do—when Delilah betrays Samson by coaxing the secret of his strength and then revealing it to those Philistines who hadn't forgiven Samson for the jawbone incidents. So they cut off his hair and beat him up, humiliating him and blinding him.

I could identify with Samson now. Bald and weak. Bereft. "It's only hair," my lover says.

"That's what Delilah told Samson," I want to say but don't.

"It will grow back," my lover says.

"If I live that long," I don't want to say but do.

"You've lost your hair, I see," the oncologist says. I could swear she's got just the tiniest smirk tainting her face as she turns to the sink to wash her hands. But when she turns back, her gaze is nothing but professional.

I want to curse her like Samson must have cursed Delilah.

Instead I ask her about my white blood counts. Low. Low. Which is the reason I feel so weak, she explains. Had I told her I felt weak? Low. Low. She frowns. But not low enough to reprieve me from another round of Adriamycin.

I try to schedule the chemotherapy on Fridays so that I can sleep and vomit all weekend and be ready to work by Monday. I'm hiding from my editor, although she doesn't seem to realize it. E-mail makes it easy, even my unsteady voice is masked by the cheery letters on the computer.

If we have to meet, I'll just wear my hat. I have a brightly colored skull cap that I'm hoping looks fashionable, especially with my new gauntness. I flatter myself that I look a bit like a model, but my illusion is shattered when a woman approaches me on the street and inquires, "Chemotherapy?" I cry and my lover nods. And the woman says, "Yes, I had it myself last year, but now I'm doing fine." I'm sure she means to be encouraging, but I feel exposed. More naked than naked.

Like Samson, on display for all the Philistines to gawk. But wait, the Bible story doesn't end there. Samson triumphs. He asks God for his strength back and God grants his prayer, and Samson pulls down the pillars of the temple where the Philistines had chained him. Killing more Philistines than he ever had before. Hooray! Samson also dies, but we are supposed to believe that his death is a small price to pay for his victory. And that what he did wasn't suicide.

I remember why I quit Sunday school.

Although I'm praying now, I'm not praying to be able to take a whole bunch of other people with me when I die, enemies or not, I don't want to smote anyone. Not even my oncologist or my editor. I only want to save myself. Please God, let my hair and my strength come back and I'll be faithful forever after.

Which is what Samson should have prayed if he was thinking clearly. And he should have been thinking clearly, even though he was being mocked. He was only bald, after all. I mean, he probably still had hair on other parts of his body. Although *The Children's Illustrated Book of Bible Stories* is not specific on this point, it seems pretty clear that Delilah only cut off the hair on his head.

This is really different from chemotherapy, which erases the hair everywhere.

I don't really miss the hair on my legs, although I wasn't one to shave them much (I came out in the 1970s after all). And the new lack of hair under my arms doesn't cause much grief.

But I've started a poem, "Requiem for Pubic Hair."

First of all, I've learned that this hair has a function—to keep one's underwear from sticking to flesh. If I haven't paid enough attention in the past to this buffer between my tenderest folds and the world, I promise I'll appreciate it in the future. Just please come back. I'm praying to the Goddess, figuring God the Father will not be very sympathetic when it comes to this.

Then there's the aesthetic factor. Sure, when I first started springing curls in my crotch, I thought it was rather ugly. At thirteen, it seemed so private and vaguely sinister, but it didn't take very long to learn to love these swirls, mirroring as they did what I found fascinating on other women. Women. Not babies or girls, but women.

The one time I did find myself in bed with a woman without pubic hair, I was appalled. My hand didn't believe what it felt, and I tried to act as if nothing was strange. When she stripped off her underpants, she stood up and spun around for my admiration. I think I asked her what happened, as if she'd suffered some injury. She told me she shaved for her boyfriend because he liked her "smooth" and "girlish." She jutted out her mons and it seemed to glow like a half moon reflecting the light coming through her window from the streetlamp. I pulled myself together and left her bed, muttering something about not doing bisexual girls. Which was a lie, Goddess forgive me. It was the hairless crotch that sapped all my sex, all my strength.

I never wanted to fuck little girls and I never wanted to be one. When I was seven I wanted to be nine. When I was twelve, I wanted to be seventeen. When I was eighteen, I wanted to be twenty. While my friends mourned and groaned, I celebrated being thirty. I felt a sense of accomplishment at being forty.

And now, I want to live to be forty-five.

Fifty.

Goddamn it, sixty, seventy, eighty.

I want to outlive my oncologist and my editor.

My oncologist thinks the chances of this are slim to none. Six months to a year, I figure, though she hasn't said this because I haven't asked. I think they train these doctors nowadays not to tell you things like that unless you ask. Here's what she does say:

"Inoperable."

"The chemotherapy has been unsuccessful."

"Radiation is not recommended."

"A difficult and aggressive rare cancer."

"There's nothing else we can do."

She suggests a psychiatrist again.

To help me deal with "it."

I don't ask what "it" is. Thankfully she doesn't tell me.

I don't tell my editor. How can I say this in a snappy e-mail: "BTW, I'm dying."

I have to write my way out of this.

I remind myself that my Sunday school teacher told me I couldn't be a dyke and that my high school English teacher told me I couldn't be a writer.

Hah!

I grew up to be a dyke writer.

So what if my oncologist is telling me I can't survive?

And so what if my editor is saying my plight isn't good copy?

I will live to tell this tale.

It's too early to close my file, Ms. Oncologist. And it's too soon to wonder whether my work might be more marketable posthumously, Ms. Editor.

I shall defy everyone again.

If only for today, this bald dyke lives.

# Bone Scan

*Sandra Steingraber*

You submit by making a fist.
This is where the long process of unlikelihood
begins.

I make mine by curling the thumb
over top of the knuckles
the way the boy in homeroom showed me
the year the bus stop threats flew so thick
my eyes blurred with fear.

The way they are now.
The way yours will be.

"Not the sissy way," he reproached,
pulling my thumb from its foolish
grip inside the four other fingers.

"You'll break a bone that way
swinging it into the bitch's face."

You begin with a fist
and then you lay the throbbing arm down
so the blue vein can rise to meet
the probing rubbery fingers.
This is how you submit
to the lead canister decaled
with red and yellow atomic flowers
as it opens now like an Easter egg.
And nested inside: the syringe.

*Make a fist, please. And release.*
*And make a fist. And release.*

There are other lessons to unlearn.
Water, for example, serves to concentrate,
speeding the isotope's uptake
into the cells of the skeleton you hadn't known
could be a sponge for such poison.
You can go where you like for this part—
back to the waiting room or to lunch
still being served in the cafeteria.
Two quarts in two hours is recommended.

Now you yourself are the X-ray,
both photographer and landscape, exposed
and exposing, your whole radioactive self
positioned under the black absorbing plates.
Teeth, ribs, sockets, the spine's
bony rope, any hard place an errant
cancer cell could latch on, wrap around,
suck onto like a barnacle on a ship's hull:

the image of your Halloween body rises
slowly into the color monitor.

Know that the unholy energy streaming
out of your bones has nothing at all
to do with you, gripped as you are
in a half-life of absolute motionlessness,
obediently breathing as lightly as possible.
Just as the pianist knows nothing
about what the page turner is thinking
during the whole long solo.

You can pass the time with meditation,
visualization. You can hope
what you want to hope.
By predetermination, someone
in the technical audience will be cruel,
talking petulantly and ceaselessly
above your head to somebody else.
She doesn't care about you.
Here is a trick: send your soul out
into the straight bones of your fingers
as they lie there, emitting and emitting.
Imagine them curling, thumb on the outside.
Imagine the fist as it comes crashing
into those teeth.

Note:
A bone scan is a method of imaging the skeleton. A bone-seeking radioactive isotope is
injected into the bloodstream and is absorbed over a two-hour period. The patient then
lies motionless on a scanner table while her bones emit gamma rays that expose a plate of
photographic film.

# Departure

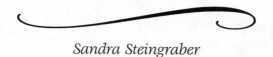

*Sandra Steingraber*

1.

For days they lifted buckets
of eels from the river. The Rhine.
*Das Gift.* The eels were dead.
From the papers we copied down numbers:
how many tankerfuls of pesticide
for how many kilometers for how many years.
About this, the old masters have no words
for us. Anger works the poison deeper
and each night the barges went on colliding.
A *departure from accepted procedures.*

2.

In Minnesota that spring, a woman
spent some days bent to a radio.
She was trying to follow the wind's path

from Kiev. When it passed over Red Wing
the cows' milk swam with cesium.
She was advised not to be concerned.
She climbed the fire tower
and scanned the clouds, watched an eagle
lift from a stand of old white pine.
She said she didn't know what
she was looking for. *An aberration.*

"Cesium 137 has a half life of 30 years."
*A freak accident.* "Cesium forms strong bonds
and sinks into the earth fractions
of inches per year." *An equipment
breakdown.* "This is how cesium
enters the grass-cow-milk route."
*Every effort is made.*

3.
We walked along the Rhine every day
for months—past the *Chemische Werke*
and the Schierstein Bridge and down by the house
where Wagner wrote *Der Meistersinger*
but where he never heard any strain of voice
descend the way cesium descends
into the bones of children. Fish ovaries
ringed with pesticide. *Wholly unpredictable.*

That was the day the American newspapers
ran the picture of the Pennsylvania treasurer
at his indictment emptying the barrel
of a gun into his mouth. *A case
of human failure.* In the cafe
by the docks the foreign workers
filed in, filed out. All morning

we turned pages, copied down numbers.
The river's head, the river's mouth.
The eels still rising.

We hoisted crates of bottled water
up the hill, the accepted procedure.
It's true, isn't it?
Every night they open the sluices.

Notes:

In November 1986, a fire in a chemical warehouse in Switzerland led to the dumping of 66,000 pounds of pesticides into the Rhine River. Under the cover of panic and confusion, other companies released toxic substances downstream. A series of mysterious shipping accidents caused the dumping of additional hazardous chemicals into the river.

In April 1986, fallout from the world's first nuclear power plant explosion in the Ukranian atomic settlement of Chernobyl covered much of Germany with a cloud of radioactive fission products such as cesium 137.

Quoted and italicized phrases are appropriated from editorials and magazine articles about Chernobyl.

*Das Gift* (German): "poison."

"The wind's path from Kiev" refers to the fall-out contaminated wind from the Chernobyl nuclear accident.

Red Wing refers to the town of Red Wing, Minnesota.

*Chemische Werke* (German): "chemical factories."

# "A Private Little Hell"
## Selected Letters of Rachel Carson

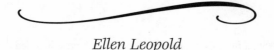

*Ellen Leopold*

RACHEL CARSON CLEARLY WOULD HAVE BEEN FORGIVEN if she had remained the well-behaved ladylike patient she was expected to be. But she was no more orthodox in her response to this terminal illness than she had been to the manmade assaults on the natural environment that had fired her scientific imagination. But as with her battles against the giant chemical corporations, she had to be selective; she couldn't challenge the established treatment of breast cancer on all fronts. It is remarkable that she managed to confront it at all. But, without ever losing her poise, she chose to reject the role of compliant patient and to become instead an advocate for herself, to be her own "case manager" in the days before such a phrase had even been coined.

It was one thing for doctors to confer or correspond with each other behind their patient's back. It was quite another for a patient to play this game herself. Carson violated the implicit confidentiality of the doctor/patient relationship (traditionally binding on the patient but not on the doctor) by reconstructing her own narrative of illness. Relying upon the clinical detachment she understood as a scientist, she pieced together a summary of her experience which she took to Dr. Crile, a man who had been her friend before he became her consultant. She wanted a second opinion and independent advice well before such things were common practice. Her direct appeal to Crile was an end run around her own doctor. Although she hadn't objected to a radical mastectomy, she *did* object to not being told the truth, or the whole truth, about the results of this surgery. More than two years later, when looking back on her ordeal with a more experienced eye, she regretted having chosen Dr. Sanderson in the first place: "How differently I would handle it now—how carefully I would select the surgeon. It's hard to see how I could have given so little thought to the possibilities." But even if her uneasiness about her doctor's response was, in the immediate aftermath of her surgery, more an apprehension than an articulated grievance, it was nonetheless sufficient to prompt her to contact Crile, generating the correspondence reproduced below.

Just how atypical Carson's response was in 1960 can be glimpsed from a breast cancer diary published in the same year. Written by a woman who described herself as a "gray-haired professor of Bible in a church-related college," it was one of the very earliest attempts by a breast cancer patient to provide a source of emotional comfort to fellow sufferers. With a foreword written by her doctor after her death, the memoir recounts anecdotes and offers advice that highlight the virtues of Christian resignation. As the author puts it, "When I first learned of the possibility of cancer, I stood on a street corner and cried inwardly, "This is too big for me to handle, Father! Please take over!" Rather than actively participating in the decision-making process, she preferred to put herself in the hands of her physicians, relieved that "God has led me to efficient doctors." Carson's response could hardly be more different. She approached her own ordeal without the comfort or conviction of religious faith, relying instead on her own clear-eyed intelligence to shepherd herself over the rocky terrain of her illness.

It's hard to imagine anyone diagnosed with breast cancer in 1960 who was more aware than Rachel Carson of the controversies surrounding both the causes of cancer and many of its treatments. Her files for the cancer chapters in *Silent Spring* show an interest in the evidence of cell damage caused by manmade chemicals used in industry and agriculture; she also kept track of the possibly harmful effects of chemicals and other substances used in cancer treatments. Just months before undergoing radiotherapy herself, Carson was clipping newspaper articles suggesting that "even small amounts of radiation may entail some risk of biological damage," that there was "no threshold dose, or dose rate, below which medical x-rays fail to cause genetic mutation." Her awareness of the risks of conventional treatment added to her well-documented suspicion of chemical companies as manufacturers of pesticides made her much more open to experimenting with alternative treatments that lay beyond the reach of the medical-industrial complex.

Carson insisted on running her public and personal lives on separate if parallel tracks, each one sealed off from the other. This old-fashioned code of conduct strikes a 1990s sensibility as extraordinary. We have grown so accustomed to first-person rather than third-person narratives of illness that the reticence of someone of Carson's generation and class now seems positively self-denying. By its absence in much of Carson's writing, we see that the first-person narrator in others' accounts serves in some way as the reader's protector and companion. When a story of illness is recounted in a contemporary memoir, the narrator takes the reader by the hand and leads her through every stage of the labyrinth of treatment, pausing along the way to share her reflections and interpretations of events. Most important, at the end of the story, she often puts the treatment behind her, living proof that there is a way out of the medical maze, back to "normal" life. Of course for Carson, there wasn't a way out. The bleaker, less modulated narrative of her experience was a reflection of her writing in active battle mode rather than in peaceful retirement.

Carson's apparent professional detachment toward her illness may suggest an impoverished emotional life to the modern reader. But though even her friends could remark on her "incapacity for chitchat," she had many close friendships. During the years of her illness, she was perhaps closest to Dorothy Freeman, a near neighbor of hers in Maine. Their letters to each other, recently published, were often warm and intimate. But their correspondence also respected a code of conduct of its own, distinguishing between letters that could be shared with other family members and letters that could not (the latter were referred to as "apples" and were sometimes folded inside the former). This unyielding sense of privacy, which valued a clear and unbridge-able separation between the public and the personal, can be hard for more modern sensibilities to grasp. Its clarity is perhaps emblematic of an earlier culture where social behavior was neatly compartmentalized, each chamber clearly defined and subject to its own set of rules.

In fact, the rigid separation of public and private experience that is built into Carson's perspective on her illness is really an accurate reflection, at the individual level, of a much more pervasive pretense that operated across soci-ety at large. The broader public refusal to acknowledge the existence or the extent of the disease or to reveal the extraordinary physical and emotional suffering it caused operated as a powerful taboo. Public denial of private an-guish added the ingredient of shame to the mix of terror and pain that the disease itself inflicted. Something so terrible that it had to be hidden away—both literally and figuratively—brought disgrace rather than compassion in its wake.

In rejecting the reality of breast cancer, society dismissed as insignificant the suffering and death of all those women who experienced it. Lying beyond the limits of the public imagination, breast cancer was virtually outlawed. Any reference to it, therefore, was a dangerous and unwelcome reminder of one's outsider status.

In this context, Carson's handling of her own situation was entirely con-sonant with the social mores of her time. She never chafed against the pre-vailing conventions. For her, breast cancer simply occupied a place in two spheres of her life. As an illness that had to be treated, it became the subject of medical attention and experiment; as a personal catastrophe, it remained strictly private, hers to consider and to control. The two were not to be confounded. Even when she was visibly suffering, she worked hard to keep her pain private. "There is no reason even to say I have not been well," she urged her friend Dorothy Freeman. "If you want or think you need give any negative report, say I had a bad time with iritis that delayed my work, but it has cleared up nicely. And that you never saw me look better. . . . I know what happens when even an inkling of the other situation gets out. As last night, scraps of dinner table conversation about poor Senator Neuberger: 'You know she had a cancer operation' . . . 'They say she's down to 85 pounds' . . . That's the sort of thing I couldn't bear and the reason I have told so few people. Whispers about a private individual might not go far; about an author-in-the-news they go like wildfire."

Although Rachel Carson was not diagnosed with breast cancer until 1960, she had had prior experience of breast disease. Fourteen years earlier, in 1946, when she was 39 years old, she had had a breast cyst removed. Four years after that, a physical checkup revealed a lump in her left breast. She knew it might turn out to be serious but approached the possibility circuitously. "There is a small cyst or tumor in one breast," she wrote to her agent Marie Rodell, "which the doctor thinks I should get rid of, and I suppose it is a good idea. . . . The operation will probably turn out to be so trivial that any dope could do it; but of course there is in such cases, always the possibility that a much more drastic procedure will prove necessary." The tumor, "about walnut-size and very deep," was removed on September 21, 1950. According to her biographer, when Carson specifically asked her surgeon whether the tissue biopsy showed any evidence of malignancy, she was told it did not. Her doctors recommended no further treatment.

While it is possible that this tumor was benign—benign forms of breast disease do often precede malignant disease—given Carson's subsequent medical history it seems most unlikely. If it was a cancer, how did the pathologist miss it? A negative finding on a biopsy is always inconclusive; it does not rule out the possibility of cancer cells in other parts of the tissue not sampled. But with no other reason to suspect a malignancy in a 43-year-old woman, perhaps the biopsy was less rigorous than it might have been. Or perhaps the whole tumor was not removed, despite what Carson had been told. With surgeons all too ready to perform radical mastectomies, it seems unlikely that the misdiagnosis, if that's what it was, was deliberate. And though it might be tempting to imagine that the earlier detection of Carson's cancer might have saved her life, the virulence that her disease displayed later on suggests otherwise. Earlier treatment might have prolonged her life but metastatic cancer would still have killed her.

In March 1960, ten years later, Carson discovered what she thought were more breast cysts. Surgery at Doctor's Hospital in Washington on April 4 revealed two tumors in her left breast, one "apparently benign," and the other "suspicious enough to require a radical mastectomy." Carson, unlike most cancer patients at the time, had actually asked her surgeon, Dr. Sanderson, whether the tumor was malignant. Whether he was prepared for such candor is not known. He certainly did not respond in the same spirit of openness but told her instead that she had "a condition bordering on malignancy." The fact that he prescribed no follow-up treatment must have reinforced Carson's understanding that there was really nothing to worry about. But less than nine months later, she came to realize that she had been deceived.

Carson must have found Dr. Sanderson's prevarication doubly galling. As a woman who had achieved remarkable success both as a scientist and a writer at a time when women were still largely excluded from public and professional life, she would have been stunned by the paternalism of her surgeon's remarks. But as a scientist, and one who paid a high price for her own integrity (in the face of opposition from the chemical industry), she might also have seen Dr. Sanderson's lie as a kind of data falsification that violated the ethics of clinical medicine as of science. She certainly tried to preserve an impartial view of her own "case"; how could her doctor fail to do so? Whatever her reaction, it was strong enough to galvanize her to get in touch with her friend Barney Crile (Dr. George Crile, Jr.) at the Cleveland Clinic.

It was a fortuitous decision. In a sense, it lifted Carson's experience of disease out of the doctor's office and created a parallel universe for it on the page, where she felt most at home. To approach Crile, she had to draw on those very skills that had already brought her so much success—a capacity for meticulous observation coupled with considerable interpretive skills. If writing gave order to her life and engendered a sense of competence, then the very act of reconstructing her own experience, however grim the details, must nevertheless have had therapeutic value for her. The clinical detachment she displays in documenting the increasing signs of terminal illness may appear to the reader as strangely dissociated, but it might have been just what Carson needed to continue her life on a business-as-usual basis, comforted by the familiarity of the process if not by its implications. That she also relied upon writing to express more intimate reactions to her ordeal is evidenced by the letters she wrote during the same period to her friend Dorothy Freeman, excerpts from which, included below, amplify the story that enfolds in her correspondence with Crile.

*December 7, 1960*
Dear Dr. Crile,

My apologies for a hand-written letter, but I've had flu and am still abed. Yesterday I tried to reach you at the clinic and learned you would return Friday, so I thought it might be as well to write you a few details, after which I shall telephone.

I hope I'm not imposing by asking your opinion on a personal medical problem but after rereading your fine book on Cancer I'm sure you can give me the advice I need on how to proceed.

Briefly, this is the story. During the past 12 years or so, I'd had two operations for breast tumors, both benign. Then last March it was discovered I had two more in the same breast. An operation was advised. The preliminary sections in the operating room aroused enough suspicion that a radical mastectomy was performed. However, the permanent sections did not reveal definite malignancy, although something was said about "changes." No follow-up with radiation was considered necessary.

All was presumably well until early November when a curious, hard swelling appeared on the 3rd or 4th rib on the operated side, at or near the junction with the sternum. At first I wasn't sure I was seeing anything, but within a week or 10 days it became obvious enough to send me to my internist and at his suggestion to my surgeon. X-ray pictures were taken and are said to show that the swelling is not the rib itself, but something lying between rib and skin. (It is, however, very hard, and not moveable.) Although both doctors acknowledge it "may" have some connection with the former trouble, they profess to be puzzled. With no further diagnostic work, they recommended x-ray therapy. The man I was referred to may be quite competent, but he does not specialize in therapy.

I had treatments last week—Nov. 28 and 29—and promptly became ill with what was first said to be either an unexpected reaction or flu. Presumably it was the latter, for I've been in bed a week with fever, aching and nausea. No more treatments, of course.

At least this has given me time to think and I now feel the whole proce-dure has been rather slap-dash in an area where that is hardly desirable! I have told the doctor (whom I've known for many years so it was easy to talk it over) that I don't want to resume these treatments at least until we have had a new evaluation of the whole thing by someone else.

Now this is where my problem lies—where my questions to you come in. What *kind* of person do you think I should see? And what kind of investiga-tion should I wish to have made in order to determine first, whether this is anything significant, and assuming it is, which of a variety of treatments would make sense? I don't want to get into the hands of an over-zealous surgeon. And I know too well that both radiation and chemotherapy are two-edged swords.

Perhaps you can make recommendations of actual names here in Wash-ington. If not, knowing the kind of person you would go to would help.

Several medically well informed people have suggested Dr. Louis Alpert, who is Medical Director of the Warwick Cancer Clinic here at George Wash-ington Hospital. Dr. Alpert himself specializes in chemotherapy. However, all types of therapy are used at the clinic and I suppose an attempt would be made to fit the treatment to the situation. However, I know the Clinic is working in chemotherapy under a grant from NIH [National Institutes of Health]—which, of course is eager to have more and more chemicals tested, and all this makes me feel just a little like a guinea pig!

I'm sure this has given you the picture and that you will understand my need of understanding advice. I want to do what must be done, but no more. After all, I still have several books to write, and can't spend the rest of my life in hospitals!!

Since I do want to see someone next week, I shall try to reach you at the Clinic Friday afternoon. Of course I shall be very grateful for your help.

Sincerely,

Rachel Carson

Carson confessed to Dorothy Freeman "that there had been pain and soreness recently quite far up in the armpit, and that I thought I felt 'something.' And I did—there is another enlarged node. It is just about on the border line of the former treatment area—would have received some radiation but not enough to prevent its going bad. Dr. C[aulk] does not want to resume immediately, and will try to wait until after my Easter trip—if I go. I'm to see him a week from Thursday and he will see how it's developing and decide.

I was quite prepared for this, as I intimated, because the pain one night was quite definite, and something new. It has not continued, but soreness has. There has also been soreness in the neck, and of course I was afraid of new trouble there, but Dr. C. says it is just the effect of treatment. So that was good news. Also, a report on the spinal X-rays showed nothing but some arthritis quite consistent with my age. I may not have told you there was some concern because my back hurt while lying on the treatment table, so Dr. C. wanted pictures. The trouble with this business is that every perfectly ordinary little ailment looks like a hobgoblin, and one lives in a little private hell until the thing is examined and found to be nothing much."

If Carson's breast cancer took her to a private hell, the publication of her book *Silent Spring* in June 1962 brought her undreamed-of public acclaim. Given the increasing pace of her symptoms, her treatments, and their side effects, it seems astonishing that she had another life at all, let alone one that required the prolonged concentration, imagination, intellectual rigor, and passionate commitment to its subject that a book like *Silent Spring* would have done. Would such an achievement have been possible if its author had not maintained such a rigid separation between her lives? As a professional woman of her generation, Carson was already quite familiar with the need to keep up a firewall between her working life and her private life: she would not have been tempted to display photographs of her loved ones on her desk at work. But her determination, like her intelligence, seems also to have been exceptional. As she put it, "It was something I believed in so deeply that there was no other course; nothing that ever happened made me even consider turning back."

Her doctors may, in some small way, have felt themselves to have been midwives to this book. They were clearly pleased to see it in print. Caulk acknowledged its publication to Crile and he responded: "It has been very satisfactory to me to know that she has been able to complete her book, and it is with great pleasure that I have been reading the installments of it currently running in the *New Yorker*."

The pain in her back did not abate. X-rays of her spine taken in December by Dr. Caulk revealed no change in her condition. When the pain failed to subside, Caulk, fearing metastases, advised five radiation sessions to her back. Crile concurred, saying that it might take two or three weeks to get the pain under control. "If it really is a metastasis, then we have gotten it quite early, before any real damage has been done. So there is much reason for optimism."

Crile's wife Jane died at the end of January, 1963, of breast cancer that had metastasized to the brain. In February, Carson's visit to Dr. Caulk revealed new lymph tumors above the collarbone, midway to the shoulder and another higher in the neck. Although Crile was reassuring, it was clear that Carson's cancer had metastasized to her bones.

*February 17, 1963*
Dear Barney,

You have been much in my mind. . . . I am glad you have the book to work on, and above all, glad you and Jane had those months to work on it together, giving it form and substance. It may be emotionally hard in some ways for you to carry it through to completion, and yet I think it will be a satisfaction.

Jane meant many things to me—a friend I loved and greatly admired, and a tower of strength in my medical problems. When she wrote me, after my visit with you two years ago, that she shared my problem, it was as though a great tide of courage flowed into me. If she, so vibrant, so gay, so full of the love of life, could live with the problem so fearlessly, I could at least try to do the same. Over the months since then the feeling I've had could best be explained by an analogy. Once, years ago, my mother and I were driving at night in uninhabited, unfamiliar country near the North Carolina coast. For the 50 or more miles through those wooded lowlands we were able to follow the lights of a car ahead. As long as it progressed smoothly I knew our way was clear. Jane was that kind of reassuring light to me. Now, without that light to follow, I admit my courage is somewhat shaken.

But you, Barney, for different reasons, are also a great source of strength. So now I'm writing you of my current problems. I didn't want to bother you while Jane was ill, and for that matter the more important ones have just happened, or at least have just been noticed.

First: I finally saw a cardiologist, Dr. Bernard Walsh, about three weeks ago. I definitely have angina (even the cardiogram is now abnormal, but he said the diagnosis was perfectly clear from symptoms alone) of the less common type in which the pains come on without physical provocation, the worst ones during sleep. Dr. Walsh said frankly the implications are serious and it is most important to get the situation under control. So—I'm virtually under house arrest, not allowed to go anywhere (except as you will see later) no stairs, no exertion of any kind. I had to rent a hospital bed for sleeping in a raised position. . . .

The second problem is in your department. About two weeks ago I noticed a tender area above the collar bone on the left (operated) side, and on exploring found several hard bodies I took to be lymph nodes. Dr. Caulk was just going out of town for several days and said he would come to the house on his return. By that time I was so sure I was going to need treatment that I just had myself taken down to see him. . . . They are definitely lymph nodes "gone bad," some lying fairly well up in the neck. This is the side opposite last year's trouble spots and is an area never previously treated. So we have begun—5-minute treatment 3 days a week to keep my hospital trips to a minimum.

Now there is a further complication. At the time I went in about my back in December I kept making remarks about having "arthritis" in my left shoulder, but no one paid much attention. It has been increasingly painful, and now there is some difficulty about certain arm movements. I had begun to have suspicions, so now I've tackled Dr. Caulk about it again. They took a picture Friday and there does seem to be trouble. He let me see the x-rays. It is the coracoid process of the scapula—the edge of it looks irregular and sort of eroded. For some reason Dr. Caulk seems rather puzzled—says he wants some of his associates to look at it and may want a picture from another angle, but on the whole he does feel it is a metastasis.

Well, all this brings questions in my own mind, which leaps to conclusions that may or may not be justified. Oh—the back trouble cleared up, but

*"A Private Little Hell"*

so slowly that Dr. Caulk had about decided it wasn't a metastasis. Treatment was begun just before Christmas and completed December 31. I was still in considerable pain in mid-January. Then rather rapid improvement set in and now it's ok. But now this bone deterioration in the shoulder makes me think all the more I had a metastasis in the spine. Dr. C. says not necessarily, but I think he's just trying to reassure me.

Barney, doesn't this all mean the disease has moved into a new phase and will now move more rapidly to its conclusion? You told me last year that it might stay in the lymph nodes for years, but that if it began going into bone, etc., that would be a different story. If this is the correct interpretation I feel I need to know. I seem to have so many matters I need to arrange and tidy up, and it is easy to feel that in such matters there is plenty of time. I still believe in the old Churchillian determination to fight each battle as it comes, ("We will fight on the beaches—" etc.) and I think a determination to win may well postpone the final battle. But still a certain amount of realism is indicated, too. So I need your honest appraisal of where I stand.

Jane continues to give me courage. Kay told me of her question to the doctors: "Which of you is in charge of not giving up?" How like her! Well, I nominate you to that post. I would like so much to discuss some of this with you, and wonder if you'd call me some day soon.

My love to the children. As ever,

Rachel

# As Luck Would Have It

*Roberta L. Hacker*

MY MOTHER ALWAYS SAID I'D BE LUCKY. It all began while she was pregnant with me. It seemed that every time she went out, a neighbor boy would ask her where she was going. She would reply, "Up in the air to get red hair." My brother, at the age of three, told my mother that he wanted a "baby sister with orange hair" for his fourth birthday. These are the legends that accompanied my birth: born on my brother's fourth birthday, a baby sister with very, very orange hair.

As far back as I can remember, there were occasions when I would *feel* my luck. When I was about seven years old, I was at a Christmas party where tickets for a door-prize drawing were distributed. As the numbers were drawn, a surge of excitement rushed through my body, followed by a tingling up and down my spine, ending with the hair on my arms feeling electrified. I felt myself slip into a parallel reality, surrounded by a slightly golden light, the voices of folks around me somewhat distant. Then, like a bolt of lightning followed by a crack of thunder, I was alert. The ticket in my hand felt hot. The next thing I knew, I was looking at my ticket—sweating as each of my numbers was announced.

As a preteen in the 1950s, I began *seeing* my luck. I won some neat prizes in three national art contests: a purebred black cocker spaniel, a nifty green and ivory girl's Columbia bicycle with a horn and headlight and a cool red and cream portable television. As I was finishing up each contest project and preparing it for submission, I would get a squirmy, excited feeling in my stomach, followed by a premonition where I would see myself winning. My father, an artist and a rather lucky guy himself, helped me with these artistic endeavors. He advised me to be patient, to let my excitement go and not dwell on dreams of winning. "Let it come to you," he would say.

Luck for me is an experience that involves a sense of strange excitement and uncanny vision. It's been this way all my life. I cannot predict when it will happen, but experiencing luck is a very visceral, physical sensation. I'm not very comfortable revealing all of this; I am afraid to "put it out there" because I don't want to jinx myself. I've always been careful not to talk too much about these experiences, which for me are magical, even mystical. And although I've had many experiences with positive luck, I've also had numerous experiences with bad luck. The feminist witch Z. Budapest said something about this being the magic of life; there must always be a balance, a positive must always offset a negative and vice versa. I've had three substantial encounters with the negative—bad luck. Each involved experiencing life as it brushed up close to death. The first incident was a motorcycle accident in October 1974; the second encounter was in October 1994, when I fell nine feet into an empty swimming pool; and the third experience was receiving my cancer diagnosis in March 1996. Each encounter profoundly changed my life as each involved both luck and mysticism.

*The Motorcycle Incident*

I was twenty-nine years old and making a career transition in social work from adult mental health to working with troubled youth. Before embarking on this new path, I planned a solo motorcycle trip from Philadelphia, Pennsylvania to Columbia, South Carolina. This was to be my first major adventure. Right before I left, I had a series of foreboding dreams filled with scenes of highway accidents, emergency rooms, permanent physical injuries and death.

I forced myself to ignore them, chalking the dreams up to anxiety about my great maiden voyage. All went well during my trip; in fact, it was extraordinary. I had no more dreams, until the last leg of my return. I stopped for the night just south of Washington, D.C., where my sleep was interrupted by several more disturbing dreams. When I began my final ride home, I made a mental note of my dreams so that I would be extra cautious. Just past Baltimore, Maryland, a car that had been pulled over on the shoulder of the highway either did not see me or did not care and began pulling onto the road in front of me. I was forced to swerve quickly and sharply to the left, struggling to maintain control of my motorcycle. I was so shaken that I pulled over to the shoulder where I sat for about thirty minutes.

When I was just about five miles from home, I stopped at a traffic light. As the light turned green, I was off. Then suddenly I saw a car heading toward me. I swerved and braked, but this time I lost control. My bike flew to the right and I flew to the left. I put my arm up to protect myself, crashing into the side of the car. I was knocked out. As I regained consciousness, I found myself lying on my back on the pavement in front of a gas station. Voices far in the distance grew louder and closer, and when I opened my eyes, I was looking up into the faces of many concerned people staring down at me.

At the emergency room the nurses said I was lucky not to have been injured more seriously. I was wearing a helmet with a face shield, several layers of clothing and gloves. Nevertheless, I had a severely shattered left arm and had to undergo three surgical procedures: the first to repair the original injury by inserting a five-inch stainless steel plate with six screws to hold my bone together; the second was reconstructive, to repair nonfusion of the bone, which involved the removal and reinsertion of the plate, taking a cup of live bone cells from my hip and placing them on the fracture site to help it regenerate; the third surgery was the final removal of the plate. It was nearly a four-year recovery process during which my anxiety and, as the feminist scholar Mary Daly would say, "dis-ease" continued. Each surgery brought renewed fear because the symbolism of my foreboding dreams had involved personal injury, hospitals and ultimately death.

While I was recovering from the reconstructive surgery, I had an incredible encounter: I awoke feeling as though someone were holding me, lying next to me with an arm across my waist. I felt warm and protected. But as sleep faded, the presence slipped away, and instead I saw before me three hooded figures. They did not invoke fear but rather warmth and love. I wanted to be with them; I begged the figures to take me with them, but they told me no, it was not yet my time. I was stunned as they disappeared into another dimension. That encounter gave me much to think about, including a way to allay my fears of loss and disability. Each time I recollected the encounter, I gained the strength to regenerate the injured parts of my body and the courage to reach out to friends and family for help and support. The confluence of my dreams and visions led me to a path of self-exploration. I began believing in my intuitions—and in luck.

### The Pool Incident

My father died in 1994. Although I was forty-nine at the time, I suddenly felt like an orphan. (My mother had died in 1989.) As I worked through my sense of loss and abandonment, I had many dream encounters with my parents. That June, I had to put my first cat, Sashay, to sleep. I nursed her for six months until her death from breast cancer. She had been a wonderful gray-and-white who found me in 1980. It had been a sad year.

On a bright fall Saturday in late October, my partner of eleven years and I took a trip to the New Jersey shore to visit her mother. Rather, she was going to visit her mother, and I was going to fly my beautiful fifty-foot dragon kite, Serpentina. I called it sky-fishing, a hobby I had pursued since childhood. I loved the dragon kite because it was gentle, magnificent and acrobatic. This day was sunny, clear and with just the right wind. I was busy putting Serpentina through her routines when I decided to send up a couple of small streamers on her line. As I was concentrating on attaching the streamers, a gust of wind grabbed Serpentina, something that had never happened to me before. I was upset and irritated. Being slightly overweight and prone to asthma attacks, I decided not to run after the kite, but to let her go. Fortunately, a land wind rather than a sea wind had taken her, so I knew the kite would be hung up somewhere not far away.

Gathering together my sky-fishing accoutrements, I made my way from the beach to the street, keeping my eye on Serpentina and trotting in the kite's direction. I saw that she had stopped not too far ahead, so I wove my way through alleys and motel parking lots until I came upon the motel where Serpentina had taken up residence. High atop a tower on the motel, Serpentina was swaying in the wind. Determined to get her back, I surveyed the area, tried to access the roof deck, to no avail, and decided to try to yank and nudge the kite down by her line. My strategy to untangle the line failed however, and I misjudged my proximity to a drained swimming pool. I fell in head first.

As I fell, I saw the nine-feet marker on the pool side. Then I hit bottom, unconscious in a foot of disgusting, stagnant water. After regaining consciousness, I stood and thought to myself, "I'm okay." I felt what I thought was water draining from my left ear, so I tried to jump and shake my head to make the water come out. That's when the pain took over, and I realized blood was pouring from my ear. I almost passed out again from the pain in my shoulder and back. I could not walk upright, so I lay down on my right side and tried to crawl from the deep end of the pool toward the steps at the shallow end. Not a chance; I was in too much pain and shock was setting in. I wanted to close my eyes and go to sleep. I was tired, wet and cold. I wanted to go to sleep and wake up to find that this had been a bad dream. But dusk was quickly approaching, and I knew I had to keep myself awake. I called for help.

It seemed like an eternity before anyone answered my call. I reached deeply into my spirit to garner enough strength to project out to my partner for help. I visualized her every time I yelled. We had prearranged for her to meet me at the spot where she had left me sky-fishing. I had to trust that she would see Serpentina in the sky like a beacon summoning her to my aide. I kept calling, repelling the fears of doom that kept trying to blanket me with sleep. Then I heard my partner calling my name. Rescue was imminent. I was evacuated by helicopter to a trauma center up the New Jersey coast.

None of it seemed real to me, except for the pain. My need for sleep was so intense, it kept pulling me back into a twilight zone. Just when I thought I had reached a resting spot, someone would call my name, instructing me not to go to sleep, telling me I had to stay awake, that I had to remain connected to reality. Even as I was rolled into the trauma center, which was bustling with activity, I struggled to stay awake. Questions were asked, procedures explained, and all I could do was go with the flow. During a brief moment of quiet, my partner's mother came and asked if she could pray over me—a miracle in itself because she had not accepted my relationship with her daughter until that moment. I figured I could use all the help I could get. I was released from the hospital the next day with a fractured collarbone. However, my entire body hurt from the trauma. I had extreme pain on the left side of my head, and I was unable to hear out of my left ear. I barely remembered the ride home, although I remember being thankful that we had just moved our bedroom from the third floor of our house to the second, right next to the bathroom.

The next day I had to begin getting my life back together. First I had to find doctors for follow-up care. Through my internist I found Dr. Karen Lyons, an ear-nose-throat specialist who provided me with the best care I had ever received. She ordered a CAT scan, which revealed a barely visible hairline fracture of my skull. Dr. Lyons told me I was lucky to be alive. Until that moment the severity of my accident hadn't registered. Her words resonated as I looked at the CAT scan film. I remembered that before I had left the house that fateful Saturday, I had found a prayer card my mother had given me many years ago. It just sort of appeared, like lost things sometimes do: They disappear and then, presto, they return. I recalled holding the card, looking at the guardian angel overseeing the children as they passed over a dangerous bridge. I had turned the card over and read the guardian angel prayer and with misty eyes recalled my mother's smiling face. Now, as I viewed the x-rays of my fractured skull, I thanked my guardian angel for saving me from yet another life-threatening experience.

The orthopedist could do little other than put me in a brace that might not heal the fracture. He offered surgery but by the time I saw him, that would have meant another bone graft, which I refused to go through. My collarbone has never fused, and the orthopedist told me it is held together by gristle, much like a chicken breast. I have a visible lump on my collarbone where the fracture bulges upward.

I was out of work for four months as I recovered from the severity of the injuries I had sustained, and my relationship sustained its own body blows during this time. I had never been dependent on my partner before; in fact, I had never been dependent on anyone before. When recovering from my motorcycle accident in 1974, I lived alone; friends had helped me after the surgeries, but I was pretty much on my own, dependent only on myself. Now I had a partner to help me, but she was caught up in her own problems. She was freaked out about the reality that my life could have been lost; she was freaked out about the responsibility she now had to shoulder. She feared having to disclose information about our relationship to people at her teaching job, as she was not out at work. I felt I had to take more care of her needs than of my own. My frustration turned to rage and then depression.

*The Cancer*

By the summer of 1995 I had recovered from the pool accident, living a full life once again. My relationship also seemed to have recovered. Then I began having signs of menopause. A relief, I thought, not to have my monthly cycle. During the magic month of October, I had menstrual spotting. I decided to see the gynecologist before the end of the year so I could maximize my major medical deductions. I procrastinated until the end of December, when I saw Dr. Cynthia Cooke, a physician known for providing good care for lesbians. Dr. Cooke suggested several possibilities for the spotting—fibroids, endometriosis or endometrial cancer but doubted the latter. She advised a laparoscopic biopsy and referred me to a surgeon she trusted, Dr. Wanda Ronner. The biopsy is a basic D and C (dilation and curettage) using a video camera probe with scissors on the end. Fairly routine, the procedure is done on an outpatient basis, so I asked my partner to accompany me. Dr. Ronner made every effort to include my partner in what was going on. She even went to the waiting area to show my partner pictures of my cervix and uterus, explaining what she had seen and done. I was impressed. Dr. Ronner explained to me that she had removed several polyps from my uterus, which she had sent to the pathology lab for examination. She said she thought everything looked okay and that the polyps were the likely cause of the bleeding, a common problem in menopausal women. Although she asserted that nothing would be conclusive until the lab results were returned, Dr. Ronner doubted there was any cause for concern.

Two weeks later I had to take a business trip for several days. Upon my return, I discovered that Dr. Ronner's office had called repeatedly and finally the doctor herself had called emphasizing that I needed to see her immediately.

Back in the examining room, I was told gently what the pathology tests had revealed: My uterus had atypical cells, meaning endometrial cancer. Dr. Ronner was totally surprised by the lab results. I felt as though I were outside of my body, far above, looking down on me and the doctor. I could faintly hear what was being said and I could hardly see, as the room was suddenly filled with a bright, blinding light. Many questions flashed through my head, most having to do with pain and death. I asked Dr. Ronner what she recommended. Given my age—fifty-one—she recommended a total hysterectomy as soon as possible. I said I needed a couple of months to get my affairs in order, and she said I didn't have a couple of months: I needed surgery immediately or the cancer would advance. The doctor explained that my hospital stay would be less than a week, and to speed my recovery, she recommended epidural anesthesia. Once home, my recovery would be about four to six weeks.

Dr. Ronner said I was lucky that Dr. Cooke had been a skilled diagnostician. Another doctor might have simply passed my symptoms off as menopausal. The laparoscopic biopsy had caught the cancer at a relatively early stage. But I didn't think I was lucky; early detection was good, but I still had cancer. As I told my partner the diagnosis, we were both upset, but I knew I had to keep myself focused and positive. I wasn't sure I could rely on my legendary luck to pull me through yet another life-threatening experience.

I can barely remember the time between the diagnosis and the day I went to the hospital. I was in that faraway place, watching as I went through the motions of preparing for surgery and possibly my own death. I tried to view this merely as a new experience, as I was prepped for surgery. I was barely conscious by the time I got to the operating room where I was greeted by Dr. Ronner. The surgery was, medically speaking, uneventful. Dr. Ronner told me she had called in an oncologist, Dr. Timothy McGuinness, who performed a very careful and thorough examination of my lymph nodes, which included more biopsies to make sure all signs of the cancer were removed. My stay in the hospital was short, only four days. On the second day the epidural was removed. My incision was only seven (a lucky number) inches wide. I was able to get up and walk around with hardly any pain. Dr. Ronner was amazed by my attitude and ability to move around. But I wanted to get better and go home; that was my goal. Before my discharge the doctor reported that all of the biopsies were negative. She reiterated that I was lucky: The cancer had been on the verge of perforating my uterus, which was why she had called in the oncologist. I was lucky, she told me, because I had what is called a "surgical resolution" of my cancer; I would need no chemo or radiation therapy. I would need close monitoring by Dr. Ronner and Dr. McGuinness for at least two years, but both were hopeful that I would have no recurrence.

My recovery at home—April through June—was relatively painless, at least physically. In July Dr. Ronner advised caution but said I could do whatever I wanted physically. As I recovered, I became very depressed, however. I wanted to believe this was because of my hysterectomy, which can cause hormonal shifts, or that it was the lingering impact of my cancer diagnosis. But it wasn't. My partner had become distant and detached, and soon I realized she was having an affair with a much younger woman. Apparently one life-threatening experience was as much as she could handle; her fears of my possible disability and death drove her to seek someone far too young to be concerned about either eventuality. My emotional trauma now superceded my physical pain.

I was so depressed that I felt seriously suicidal; I cried constantly. I had survived cancer surgery but now was threatened with the loss of my partner of thirteen (an unlucky number) years. By mid-July I had begun therapy with Dr. Ruth Steinman, who diagnosed me with clinical depression, likely a result of a chemical imbalance in my brain caused by my head injury. She prescribed Zoloft. Soon the fog lifted and I felt more in control of my emotions. I had survived the surgery and even the dissolution of my relationship. Now I had to regain control of my life.

The next few months were among the most painful of my life, more terrifying than the cancer, more destructive than my previous serious accidents. I confronted my partner, but we were unable to resolve our problems. The best solution was for her to move out, which she did in September, fewer than five months after my cancer diagnosis. The rest of 1996 I spent grieving the many losses I had suffered over the past few years and strategizing about how I would rebuild my life. The irony of survival is that fear lingers. I know that I have been lucky to have survived several life-threatening situations, and survival has made me cautious. I no longer ride a motorcycle; there are no crashes in my future. I still fly my kite, but I won't be climbing any motel towers again and doubt I'll have a second cataclysmic fall into another empty pool. These accidents threatened my life and left their scars—both physical and emotional—but I survived. My physical injuries have healed; even my emotional injuries from the loss of my partner will heal. There was an end to my recovery from those accidents, and I know the wound left by the severing of my relationship will also heal. These things are finite.

Cancer is infinite, however, at least until it kills you. It lurks and hovers, like the evil twin of the guardian angel on the bridge who protects you against danger. Cancer *is* danger, unseen, like the car coming out of nowhere as you turn on your motorcycle, or the one false step backward as you look skyward toward a kite. Cancer is the endless accident, the continual fall. It has no end, at least no end that you can depend on.

I know I am lucky, because everyone tells me I am. And the truth is, I *am* lucky. But the unpredictability of cancer leaves me unsettled. After surviving so much, after having been broken and healed and broken and healed again, cancer has made me question my luck. Yes, I have survived; yes, I am lucky. *But for how long?*

# Vibrator Party

*Tee A. Corinne*

"Come on Ali. Don't you want to go just a little bit? Just to see what it's like?" Dale fiddled with the remnants of her croissant, eyes twinkling under her dark eyebrows, auburn hair curling just above the top of her collar.

"A vibrator party? Doing it with other people around? I don't think I could." Ali brought the coffee pot over and filled both mugs, savoring the smell. She looked at her friend, who glowed in a splash of morning sunlight. "No. I just don't think I could." She shook her head as she spoke, replacing the pot on the burner. Moving into the sunlight, she massaged Dale's shoulders through her plaid shirt. Those muscles were always tight from work and enthusiasm. "How many people did you say were invited?"

"Twenty." Dale stirred the coffee to cool it, raised the cup and inhaled deeply. "You make the best coffee in town."

"It's the cinnamon, I always tell you. You could add it to your own at home." She presses deeply with her thumbs.

"The scenery's better here. Anyway, about the party, you have to bring food to share and, of course, your own vibrator. And a towel for the hot tub."

"Hot tub? I haven't been in a hot tub with anyone around since, well, you know, since the surgery." Ali worked her way down Dale's backbone and under her shoulder blades. "And what would I do about clothing during the—would you call it 'sex' time?"

"I'm calling it an orgy and you could leave them on. Why don't you wear a tee shirt in the hot tub if you don't want people to see. Lots of the women who'll be there know about your operation. They won't mind. And if they do, it's their own problem." She drank some coffee then leaned back into Ali's fingers.

"You're serious about this, aren't you?"

"You bet, pal. You've been a turtle for far too long. I remember the days when you had a new lover every year and a few extras in between, like for special occasions. You liked sex and you liked variety." Dale's hand stroked the warm mug. "Then, when they told you that you had cancer, you quit, cold. That was it." She took another long drink.

"But my body was so pretty then, Dale. It's not any more." Ali refilled Dale's cup then leaned against the counter.

Dale's eyes held her. "Your insides are pretty. That's what people always like about you. And you're brave, too, always have been. Where's the woman who used to jump out of planes with me? Who surfed with me when we were in college? Who learned hang gliding when she was forty?"

"She's forty-five and missing some of her chest and very self-conscious. That's where she is." Ali felt herself drawing back. She crossed her arms against her friend. "Don't you understand? I'm afraid I'll make people sick. I'll ruin the party just by being there."

Ali turned abruptly to the sink and splashed cold water on her face. She was shaking. She wanted to go to the party. It was just . . . she was so afraid. She dried her face, picked up her well-cooled coffee and sat down. The sun had moved a bit. Its warmth felt good against the cold inside her.

"It's not a gathering of tender shoots, you know. We all have to deal with changes in our bodies. Some of us just have scars that don't show." Dale looked out the window, her jaw tight.

Ali remembered Dale telling of the beatings her father gave her as a kid, strapping her with a belt, calling it discipline. And those beatings had left marks inside. Dale never let anyone get very close. Ali had known her a long time and knew that those barriers were dense. She reached across and covered Dale's hand with her own.

"I know, hon. Something's hard for everyone. It's just that sex was always easy for me. Now, I feel like I have to learn all over again and maybe," she took a long drink, "maybe, it's so hard, it's just not worth it."

"Try it, you might like it," Dale said with a growl and a leer.

Ali laughed. "Okay. Okay. I'll think about it."


Arriving a little late for the party, Ali hoped she looked calmer than she felt.

"I'm still not sure this is a good thing to do." Ali carried a bag containing smoked oysters, miniature corn, olives, pickles, paté, and crackers, and her overnight case. Dale had both sleeping bags, pillows, and a knapsack. Ali glanced at her as they climbed the stairs into the old Victorian. She would be brave for herself as well as for Dale. She didn't have to do anything she didn't want to. She could hang out in the kitchen or watch videos or climb into her sleeping bag and go to sleep. Sleep? Would she be able to sleep, or, if she participated, would she be able to climax? Hell, could she even plug it in? Could she bear to look at other women with both their breasts?

She rang the bell.

"Welcome." Lena, smiling warmly, swung the door wide wearing a flowery, elegant caftan. Her hair a pale pink-orange spray around her head. "Settle your gear in the third room on the left. The kitchen's on down the hall. Hot tub's out back."

Shortly, Ali sat in what must have once been a bedroom. Now the floor was covered wall-to-wall with foam pads topped by patterned rugs. Electrical outlets were prominent above the baseboards. Lighting was low. On the walls were enlargements of old pornographic pictures, pastel tinted views of women together in and out of turn-of-the-century garb. Ali had seen their like before but always small, in books. She stared now, wondering what the women's lives had been like. Were they happy? Well-paid? What happened when they reached middle age? She wished some of them had scars.

"Hi, pal. Dreaming?" Dale, wearing a terry robe, leaned against the door.

"I used to look like that, only skinnier. I wish I'd had some pictures taken. You know, before." Ali finished unrolling her sleeping bag, then took her vibrator and abruptly plugged it into the nearest socket. Turning to her friend, she raised her chin and took a deep breath.

"Dale . . . "

"You're doing fine, pal, just fine. And looking great. No one can tell if the glitter in your eyes is terror or excitement."

A recording of *We've Come A Long, Long Way* played in the distance. It was true she'd come a long, long way. Just getting this far, to this house, this room, had taken so much. Could she go that further distance to the hot tub and, beyond that, party later in this room?

She undressed down to a tank top that said IT'S A NATURAL, put on her kimono and followed Dale down the hall, her heart banging around as if her chest were hollow.

"Dale, I'm just not sure." She pulled at the back of her friend's robe.

Turning, Dale gathered her into her arms, snug but not tight.

"Here. Rest a minute. We can go as slow as you like."

Ali's face pressed against the soft, worn robe. She inhaled the fresh, minty smell, the soap and cologne smells, inhaled safety, familiarity.

"Hey, you two, since when were you an item?" Joani slapped Dale on the butt, squeezed Ali's arm. "I'm jealous." Ali stared at Joani's ample body, unclothed and unmarked.

"We're not," Dale said. There was a flatness in her voice. Joani was one of Dale's ex-lovers.

"Well, well, who knows what's next?" Joani waved and headed into the bathroom.

Ali laughed, feeling the tension wash out of her. She'd known Dale longer than anyone else in her life now.

"God, we've been friends for more than thirty years!"

"I know. I don't think about it much. Makes me think I'm older than I feel." Dale put her arm around Ali in a protective way, encouraging her down the hall, staying beside her out onto the deck where all Ali could see was flesh and more flesh. Panic. Women stretched out sunbathing, giving and receiving back rubs, playing ping-pong. No one had a stitch on.

"I wish I wore glasses so I could take them off," she muttered.

Slowly her fear subsided as she recognized most of the faces even though she couldn't put names to them all. Several people waved.

"Hi, Dale."

"Hi, Ali."

"There's juice and wine on the table. Don't pee in the tub."

"Ah, there you are." Lena was submerged with several other women in the large redwood tub. She climbed out, wrapping a large towel around her waist. Ali's breath caught midway down her throat. All she could see was Lena's chest with its one full, tanned breast and the flattened curve where the other had once been, the smoothness divided by a pale, uneven scar.

With great effort Ali raised her eyes to Lena's face.

"How did you learn to be so open about . . . so calm about . . . ?" Her eyes dropped their question to the scarred line. "I've never seen anyone else's." Her hand rose and fell back.

"Do you want to touch?"

The world seemed absolutely still and very bright. The ping-pong ball resounded hollowly. A plane dully roared overhead. A yellow jacket buzzed Ali's face. Absently she waved it away.

Her pulse was very loud inside her.

Ali searched Lena's face for any hesitation and found there a quiet strength, passive, waiting.

"Yes I do want to touch." She raised her hand and lightly stroked the warm flesh, tracing the seam from end to end, then resting the back of her hand against it.

She smiled at Lena. "You're very brave."

"Arrogant too. I decided I didn't want to be cut off from my own life, from so many of the things I enjoy. My first time at a nude beach was hard, but no one paid very much attention."

Dale squeezed her shoulder. "I'm going to get some juice. Want anything?"

"Some wine with, I don't know, maybe a strawberry or something."

All around her conversations were continuing. Ali felt hot all over. Her own fear was a sharp odor in her nostrils, fear and something else . . . excitement?

Quickly she dropped her kimono and pulled the tank top over her head.

"So yours run that way." Lena traced the dual lines inward. "When?"

"Two years ago."

Lena nodded as if taking in the whole complex surrounding the operation: the worry and anger, the sense of loss and mutilation, the shame.

"Any recurrence?"

"None so far."

Dale came back with two plastic glasses, cherries and raspberries in the light wine.

Ali took the cup, her hand shaking slightly. "Did you know this would happen?"

"I knew nothing would change if you stayed at home, old pal." Dale quickly brushed her fingers across Ali's lips and cheek.

"Come. Join us." Lena gestured toward the tub.

Ali turned and began the long, celebratory walk across the deck, Lena on one side, Dale on the other.

A murmur of voices, sighs, and groans hovered around the room, mingling with recorded music, with the smell of flowers, of musk.

Indistinct figures moved in the gentle, warm light, sometimes crossing the video screen on which two women were going down on each other.

Ali exhaled an exasperated sigh. "I just can't come." She turned off the Hatachi's motor and shifted her position, smoothing her maroon nightgown.

Dale, half-tucked into a sleeping bag next to her, clicked off her antiquated Oster and turned from the video.

"Want some help, pal?"

"Or some from me?" Lena, her loose robe open, knelt beside Ali, a tin of oysters in her hand. "Here, try one of these."

Ali ate without thinking, then focused on the warm, heavy flavor, eating from Lena's fingers, sucking the juice. The buttery, smoky smell reminded her of being a child at adult parties, sampling the hors d'oeuvres. It was a welcome and comforting memory.

Lena spread the oil across Ali's lips, leaned down and kissed her, then fed her another oyster and ate one herself. "Help? Yes?"

"Yes." Ali nested into the pillows, felt Dale's arm behind her head. Lena's hand stroked her belly through its satiny covering, pushing and kneading the touch-hungry flesh. Lena smelled like summer gardens back home, long ago. Ali breathed the scent in, softened into it, into her friends' arms.

Tingling sensations began to spread from Ali's twat down along her legs, upward to where her breasts had once been and beyond. She took the Hatachi in her hands again and thumbed the switch.

Everything intensified.

Lena leaned over and touched her lips with the taste of oysters followed by soft lips, touching, parting, a fine hard tongue, caressing.

She felt warm hands moving along her legs, squeezing and molding her body, thawing her fear.

Ali moaned into Lena's lips. How could anyone touch her like that? How did she know just what was needed and give just that, no more?

Dale's body cradled her from behind, cradled and rocked her slightly, rocked against her.

Doors, long shut, opened inside her.

Ali rotated the Hatachi, pulsing with its insistent drone. She knew she'd have to work for this orgasm, to reach for it, to leap into it, trusting that her newest and oldest friends would hold onto her, that their loving, like a parachute, would break her fall.

Thrusting against the Hatachi, she felt the tensions building, the climax gathering. She willed herself to the brink, to finally let go, like jumping from a plane, pushing herself forward even when something in her said no, no! Bringing herself to the brink again, longing for that rush of exhilaration, the wind in her hair.

Surely letting go here was safer than the many jumps she'd made before, surely.

Dale spoke words of loving encouragement in her ear. Lena's hand kept up a slow, massaging rhythm, steady, non-obtrusive.

Mentally Ali imagined jumping. Opening herself to all her feelings, she opened her mouth to Lena's lips, her awareness to Dale's support.

She opened her spirit.

Lena's hand caressed her scars.

As Ali moved against the vibrator, her whole body seemed to go into motion. Her hips, shoulders, and head moved. Her legs and feet moved against each other. She courted pleasure, welcomed it through her skin and muscles, into her bones and psyche.

Warmth broke across her, flooding her. She felt the pain as well as the pleasure of climax, the orgasm wrenched from some tightly held knot deep inside her, spilling and flowing. She heard herself cry out as if it were a stranger's call, a strange call, yet familiar and oh, so dear. She lost herself in the soft, enveloping warmth, bathed in it, melted into it. Time passed. She relaxed and slept.

In the morning she woke to find her face pressed against Lena's chest, her hand hugging Lena to her.

"I want to make love to you," Ali said.

"Over and over," was Lena's reply. "Over and over."

# FITTING LESBIANS INTO
# BREAST CANCER ACTIVISM
## An Interview with Dr. Susan Love

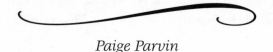

*Paige Parvin*

FOR MILLIONS OF WOMEN, the name Dr. Susan Love is synonymous with breast cancer—and she would likely consider that a compliment. Renowned surgeon, advocate, author of "Dr. Susan Love's Breast Book" and "Hormone Book," and founder of the National Breast Cancer Coalition, Dr. Love modestly calls herself a "catalyst" for sparking a new national focus on the disease and help- ing secure millions in funding for research and treatment.

Last week [In October 1999] Dr. Love visited Atlanta to speak at a lun- cheon benefiting the Wellness Community, a comprehensive support program for cancer patients. In her talk, she described an early detection screen she hopes to develop, and her full-service web-site where women can find every- thing they need to know about breast cancer, scheduled to go live in early November.

Before joining a room full of breast cancer survivors to offer words of wisdom

---

Reprinted with permission from *Southern Voice*, Atlanta's gay and lesbian newspaper.

and encouragement—as well as humor—she spoke with *Southern Voice* about her past efforts and her hopes for the future.

**Southern Voice:** Some studies seem to indicate that lesbians are at increased risk for breast cancer. In your experience, is this true?

**Dr. Susan Love:** Well, they're not exactly studies per se. . . . They take the risk factors for breast cancer, look at some of the characteristics of the lesbian population, and if you play with the math, you will come up with the conclusion that one out of three lesbians will get breast cancer. But in fact there's a whole lot of guesses in there because most of the data about lesbians was found in bars in the '50s and '60s, which doesn't really represent the majority of lesbians today, so it's not really clear.

There's certainly the same risk, and maybe slightly higher, because they don't tend to have children, and early pregnancy is a help. But it goes both ways, people get married, have children, then decide they're lesbian, and also not everybody identifies themselves, so it's tricky. The really good thing about all this is, big national studies are now asking the question about sexual orientation, so hopefully we will begin to collect data that will answer these questions.

**SoVo:** Do you feel that lesbian health is an area of women's health that warrants its own kind of attention and care, or is lesbian health sufficiently addressed in women's health care?

**Dr. Love:** It certainly warrants attention, and the question that we haven't really answered is, are there different health risks, or not? I think it's hard to characterize it as, all lesbians do everything this way all the time, therefore there are health consequences.

The biggest issues seem to be problems within the health care industry. Lesbians tend not to get regular mammograms and pap smears because they're afraid to go to the doctor, and get asked about birth control and all those issues. For most heterosexual women, the major driver is birth control, so if you're not going for birth control, then it's much easier to put it off for a few years.

So I think that what we see is less access to health care, because of lesbians' experiences with prejudice and their fears about that. Homophobia is the biggest risk for lesbians.

**SoVo:** It has been said that one reason breast cancer has not received the same kind of media attention and government funding as the AIDS epidemic is that activists have not "taken it to the streets" in the same way as groups like the controversial ACT UP. Is there a place or a need for radical activism to demand funding for breast cancer research?

**Dr. Love:** I would argue that we have taken it to the streets, with the National Breast Cancer Coalition, and some of the other groups. We're women, so we're never going to be quite as weird as the guys are. We're always better behaved, but we have been compared to ACT UP.

We now have, from $90 million, over $400 million allocated for breast cancer research. We have breast cancer activists on review committees. . . . Breast cancer has actually been one of the most successful patient lobbies ever. The Breast Cancer Coalition started in '91, so I would argue that we did take it to the streets, maybe not in the same way the boys did, but, we're girls, so we had to do it in our way.

**SoVo:** It has also been said that while lesbians were among the first AIDS activists, gay men have not come to the side of women with breast cancer in the same way.

**Dr. Love:** I think, to be totally honest, that it's a little bit of an artificial thing. I almost feel like lesbians were there for the guys with AIDS, and then they felt like it was payback time, but they didn't really have a disease to get paid back with.

And so then when the data came out, the study suggesting maybe there was a higher risk for breast cancer, everyone said, "Oh! that's our disease, we'll make that our AIDS." And it really isn't, it's not an infectious disease, it's a very different disease, and it's not as deadly. I don't know that they're totally comparable.

Then there's the argument that we helped them, and they're not helping us, but I think it's a mixed thing. It happens with the gay community. Lesbians have more in common with other women's groups than they do with gay men, so it's somewhat artificial to put the two together. What lesbians and gay men have in common is prejudice and discrimination, but in terms of how they approach the world and think and act, you see that in all the large organizations, there is a tension. . . . I'm not sure that we can expect solidarity.

**SoVo:** As a physician and a lesbian, have you found that treating lesbians for breast cancer is a different experience from treating heterosexual women? And, how do you feel lesbians are accepted in breast cancer advocacy and support groups? Do you feel there is a need for separate organizations?

**Dr. Love:** First, I don't find that it's much different as a physician. I'm sufficiently 'out' that I find it pretty comfortable either way. I do think there is a certain level of comfort for patients who are gay, knowing that that's not going to be an issue for their physician.

Ideally, everybody would like their support to be formed of people exactly like them, straight or gay, you know, or they want everybody in their support group to be 35 with two young kids and breast cancer on the left. In that sense, there's some advantage to having different groups.

But I also think there's a big advantage to realizing that there are commonalities that go across, no matter what your age, what your personal situation is. As long as it's a well-run group, and people are open and respectful of everybody else, I think it doesn't have to be segregated. But there's probably a place for both [lesbian and heterosexual support groups].

The person who really gets the short shrift, I think, is the partner of the lesbian with breast cancer. Because there's some recognition now that the men need some support, but there's really very little acknowledgement that the lesbian has a partner, and that she needs support. She can't really go to a men's support group, and she's not really welcome to the breast cancer support groups so she doesn't have that, so that's the person who I really worry about. She's a little bit in limbo and could use some support.

The other area is, sometimes lesbians or lesbian couples don't have as much family support. Sometimes you "come out" and your family disowns you, and it's fine as long as you're just going along living. But if you get breast cancer, it's not like you have your mother and your sister and your family around to support you, so you really need to find a community of friends.

**SoVo:** You have been credited with changing the face of breast cancer advocacy in the last decade. . . .

**Dr. Love:** Well, millions of women have been involved with that. I feel more like I am a catalyst. I am somebody who's not afraid to speak up and say what needs to be done.

*SoVo:* So, what's next? Will breast cancer remain your focus?

**Dr. Love:** This is definitely remaining my focus, but it's expanding to include menopause and midlife women. As baby boomers are getting older, there are a lot of issues around menopause.

I actually have a web-site coming up . . . It will be focused on breast cancer and midlife women. What we're hoping is to really set the standard for medical information on the web because what I see is very superficial information.

What most people do is take the information that's in print and just put it up there, they don't take advantage of what you can do with web technology, both in terms of interactive stuff, and in terms of allowing people to track any way they want. If you're reading a book, the author decides the order the topics should be in, but on the web, you can go to something and that can peak your interest, and you can track right over there, then back. . . .

Another advantage of the web is you can build a whole community with book reviews, columns, op ed pieces, me blasting off my opinions, and if there's something in the news, you can come right on the site and get another perspective on it.

And, this is an advantage, the web is where you could have a support group for lesbians with cancer. You could have all these isolated rural lesbians who are never going to be able to pull together a support group in their town, or maybe don't want to come out, and yet could log on to a support group on the web. That's where you can really start to do it because you have such a large population. So I'm hoping it will allow all those kinds of things.

I'm also hoping that in a subversive way, it will improve health care in America. If you give women good information on what they should be doing, current guidelines and standards, they can then go back and look at what their doctor is telling them, and ask questions, and in a lot of ways that forces their doctor to keep up.

And sometimes all you need is somebody to say, "No, being treated like that is not okay." You need to demand to be treated well. It's another way to change the world.

Dr. Susan Love's web-site: www.SusanLoveMD.com

# SELF-EXAMINATION
### (in memory of Sally Saeko Oikawa)

### Mona Oikawa

Crimson fades to brown.
My blood ritual turns softly,
gently ending.

I am afraid.

Will this month
I place my hands
in their positions?
One hand under head,
the other to wander
over breast and nipple.
Then repeat,
fingering firmly
the other one.

One.
Like my mother's one
where once were two.
One.
Like the doctor's cut of
one, just one,
assuring,
"Your mother's childbearing years are over.
She doesn't need it anymore."

I open the pamphlet,
read for the hundredth time.
"Stand in front of mirror
Raise both hands above your head.
Look for puckering, discoloring, inverting . . . "

I am doing it wrong.
I will go to the doctor
next month.

I lie on my bed.
Waiting.
In full daylight
it feels safer than at night.

Unclothed
my body opens
beneath my hands.
Memories help cleanse away
the fear.

I think of the women,
lovers who have loved
my breasts

not hesitant in
their exploration.

I want someone on me now:
A woman's mouth
sucking me hard,
making me hot with life,
tongue-teasing me to scream,
to fill this moment with
craving rage
instead of silent grief.

Mourning the loss of
my mother's breast,
my mother's life.

# Handling Your Tumor
# with Knowledge and Humor

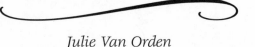

*Julie Van Orden*

I KNEW THE INSTANT I FELT THE LUMP that I had cancer. Most people, including my partner at the time and the surgeon who eventually biopsied the lump, felt I was overreacting. The surgeon said, "It will take me forty-five minutes to cut it out and tell you it's benign." Others offered statistics: "Eighty percent of breast lumps are not cancerous—it's probably nothing." So I dragged my heels making medical appointments. (Lesson One: *Never* discount your intuition. Make that appointment.)

Checkup time—finally! The gynecologist decided that my breast lump should be aspirated, which means the doctor pokes a needle into the lump to see if any fluid can be drawn from it. If there's fluid drawn, that usually means the lump is only a benign fluid-filled cyst. "It's solid," says the gynecologist. "It needs to come out, *now*, regardless of what it is." Transfer from kindly gynecologist to nasty surgeon. An episode of painful cutting (not enough anesthesia). A quick delivery of the excised material to the pathology lab (the surgeon decided he didn't like the way it looked). A phone call back to the operating room five to ten minutes later. "It's cancer," the doctor announced.

Probably unable to cope with his own stupidity, he left the room abruptly without another word.

How could a doctor have treated a breast lump so lightly when breast cancer is practically epidemic, and then, after finding out it's cancer, deliver the bad news to the patient and waltz out without so much as a consoling word? (Lesson Two: If you, as a patient, *ever* get a reaction like this, get a new doctor—immediately! Ask for a consultation from your new doctor, not a second opinion. Insurance carriers may not pay for second opinions if they deem them not medically necessary.)

After the surgeon left the room (I watched in shock, not believing anyone could be so callous), I didn't know whether I was going to faint or throw up. I sincerely hoped I wouldn't faint and then throw up. I did neither. The scrub nurse (bless her heart as big as Texas) grabbed me and held on tight. I was then in shock at the compassion a nurse could feel for a total stranger. "This is not a death sentence," she said. "You have options." I heard, but I don't think I responded. She also promised to be with me during the ordeal to come. She kept her promise. Although not common practice, she managed to be elected the scrub nurse for the mastectomy and visited me in the hospital. She even called me or visited for the next couple of years to check on my progress. An extraordinary lady!

After the biopsy, I went looking for a new doctor, and I think I have never made a better decision. I found a kind, ruddy-cheeked man with sparkling eyes and an easy smile, who hugged me the minute he met me. (Lesson Three: Never allow yourself to be treated as if you don't matter. There are still surgeons out there who have a heart.)

My anesthesiologist was supposed to work miracles. He looked like Jesus Christ, which couldn't hurt. Never having been in the hospital before, I was scared stiff. He sensed this and told the nurses to give me something to relax me. Relaxed is an understatement. It gave me what I call retrograde amnesia. Apparently I was awake and alert on the way to the operating room. I even joked with my surgical team, saying that I was keeping all my friends abreast of the situation and that double-breasted jackets were no longer a Christmas gift option. They kidded me, saying I was the first "lie-down comic" they had known.

That was all told to me later—I had absolutely no recollection of it. The last thing I did remember was the nurse in the prep room asking me if I would like her to make me an origami pig. I said sure. The operation went very smoothly, and thanks to Jesus, the anesthesiologist, I woke up hungry and with no nausea. And not only was there an origami pig to greet me, but a swan, too. Well, I knew I was special then (those origami animals find a special spot on my Christmas tree every year).

I was surprised that I felt as little discomfort as I did during recovery. I was back playing tennis in nine days. The physical distress was the easy part. I was in the prime of my life, a dedicated athlete in the peak of health, and I was only thirty-four years old. The inevitable question came up: How could this have happened? Why me? I never used drugs, never smoked, drank lightly, wasn't overweight—I'm too young! Sure, I skipped a few meals, probably had too much fat in my diet, ate red meat and drank coffee, but, still, why?

My response to problem solving has always been to learn—read, study, ask questions, read some more—learn, learn, learn. I found I had two minor risk factors: An aunt on my mother's side had died of cancer, and I hadn't had a baby before I was thirty (not at all for that matter). Perhaps a combination of genetics and nature's "use it or lose it" mentality had nailed me.

Support from friends and family was overwhelming. The phone never stopped ringing. I finally gave up answering it and sat there smiling and/or crying while listening to all the wonderful messages. It was the swimming pool of illnesses (you don't know how many friends you have 'til you get one). But still, the depression came (algae in the swimming pool).

Depression—nothing I had ever heard about it prepared me for the depths to which I was about to sink. Understand that normally I am a very upbeat person, positive and confident. There was nothing positive here. The black pit is what I called it, and I was surprised to hear others describe it in a similar fashion, always using the color black. Total hopelessness and despair, a narrow, deep well with no light.

I would start by feeling a little blue. As decisions needed to be made and daily life maintained, I would start to feel overwhelmed. I would sink deeper into the pit. I would try to explain this to others, but they couldn't understand (you can't unless you've been there). They would try the "snap out of it" or "pull yourself up by the bootstraps" approach. Then I felt isolated, and that's when the walls would start to close in. Nothing would work. I couldn't make simple decisions. The effort of trying to force those decisions fatigued me so greatly I would finally sink to my knees wherever I happened to be at the time. I was totally and utterly defeated.

I would cry—not a sobbing, sweet-sorrow sort of crying, but screams of anguish and grief. All the emotions I had kept bottled up for everyone else's benefit (to appear strong and capable) were fully fermented and pressuring the cork. They were cries of betrayal and treason, humility and defeat, and total confusion. Even death looked like a better option in the face of this emotional torrent. Eyes swollen, throat raw, I would climb into bed and stay there until the feeling lessened. My personal savior was a triple shot mocha (bless you, Starbucks). If I could just drag myself out of bed and to the coffee shop, the combination of coffee and chocolate (I believe) chemically altered my depressed state enough so that I could begin to function and eventually get back to normal.

I found I couldn't lean on anyone or ask for the support I needed. I'd always been a very independent person, and I inherently knew I could wear my friends out with this depression stuff if I leaned on any one of them too hard. The only person I confided in was my new partner. She tried, I think, but eventually couldn't or wouldn't be supportive. She was too busy wallowing in guilt and self-loathing. She had left her husband of fifteen years and despised being gay. Her problems wound her tighter and tighter until she snapped one day and finally went for help. Too late for us though.

My parents had been nothing but wonderful to me, a true blessing, but I decided they didn't deserve to witness this anguish and pain. Mom would have done anything to help me, but I knew how hard the whole ordeal had been on her already. She suffered as only a mother can knowing I had cancer. As bad as I felt, I couldn't bring any more sorrow into her life. Even so, my parents did help, just by being as wonderful as they had always been, and although it wasn't a quick fix, in the long run I know it helped. I knew that if I had called, they would have come.

Support groups, therapy—people pushed me to get help. I couldn't do it. How could a therapist really care? Maybe I should have gone, I don't know, but for two and a half years I waged war with my mind. My emotions and my intellect were at odds. Emotionally I was ruined, deep in depression. Intellectually, I couldn't understand my depression. My prognosis was good: nodes negative, only 10 percent chance of recurrence—7 percent if I took tamoxifen. I should have felt good. So what if I was a little lopsided.

I chose to take tamoxifen, an estrogen blocker. It is just one more weapon in a growing arsenal against breast cancer. My particular kind of cancer really liked the estrogen I produced—bonded with it you might say. Tamoxifen blocks or disguises the estrogen receptors on cells so that the estrogen can't recognize the receptors and attach itself to the cell, thus inhibiting growth. Unfortunately, the disguise works so well that the estrogen can't find the receptors in the rest of the body either. The result is quite often a chemically induced menopause. The side effects range from hot flashes, frequent urination and vaginal itching and dryness to nausea, dizziness and, if you're lucky, the cessation of menstruation (a side effect I was enthusiastically looking forward to but never had the satisfaction of experiencing).

Another side effect can be depression. Supposedly only a small number of women experience this, but, hey, my breast lump sneaked into the small-percentage category (remember, 80 percent are benign), so why not be one of the small percentage of tamoxifen users who get depressed? Anyway, robbing a woman's body of the effects of estrogen can really trash the psyche. My body and mind eventually adjusted to tamoxifen, but I'm sure it had magnified, if not caused, my depression.

A new and understanding partner helped tremendously. Just knowing I could have a loving hug when I needed it was a priceless asset. Here was the intimate support I knew would help and had needed since shortly after surgery. Is it weakness to depend so heavily on a lover to drag you from the depths of depression? If so, I'm weak, but I'm also happy and healthy again. The cancer was cut out and is gone, as far as I'm concerned. It was the residual depression that was the real enemy. It came far closer to killing me than the cancer ever did.

I know a little something about my own mind and body and how they interact. In college I took some pre-med courses and many psychology classes, including physiological psychology. Fascinating stuff! Everyone should know a little about the body and the mind. I mentioned that, early on, I couldn't intellectually understand my depression. Well, later, I did go back to my books and notes and devise a theory of what had happened to me. It was the first step in getting better, understanding what my brain was going through physiologically.

From the time you are born (maybe even before), the brain is busy developing neurological pathways to enable you to function normally without having to think about every movement. As a child, you struggled to take that first step, you teetered, maybe fell, balanced and tried again. Such an effort for such simple movement is inconceivable to most adults. By adulthood, the path from the brain to the legs has become a veritable superhighway with neurological impulses traveling at lightning speed.

Problem solving, coping and decision making undergo a similar neurological process, and again you have a number of pathways creating behavior and personality. These, I believe, are more complex and fragile, like a maze, but the more you work your way through the maze, the more adept you become at ending up in the right place. Consider emotional trauma to be like an earthquake to that maze. It can tumble structures that took years to build and can block the pathways with the resulting rubble. A simple decision-making process, like "What shall I wear today?" can become a frustrating ordeal in which you stare blankly at your closet and end up being overwhelmed and going back to bed. Better not to wear anything than suffer the agonizing task of rebuilding those stupid mazes and pathways. After all, it took more than thirty years to build them; how do you repair them in a matter of months? You don't. You take your time (if your diagnosis has given you this luxury) and you enlist help anywhere you can find it.

Read and learn about yourself, your body, your mind, your disease. Bernie Siegel, doctor and author, counsels, "Your disease can cure you." And knowledge is the weapon with which to fight your disease. You must first know that you have cancer. Usually and unfortunately, that is the only knowledge that can motivate you to learn. Once you're motivated you can learn about the disease, about being sick, and about being healthy, emotionally and physically. Learn about Western medicine, Eastern medicine, nutrition, the healing power of the mind. Use your faith (if you have one) or a partner's love. Consider visualization. (Lesson Four: Don't close your mind to any possible ways of healing.)

I had always been taught to "look for the silver lining," and even in my experience with cancer and depression, I have found one or two. First, I feel fortunate to have been given, as they say, a second chance. I am a lot nicer to my body. It gets all sorts of minerals and vitamins and antioxidants. I have learned about the tremendous value of nutrition, and I feel better than I did before I was diagnosed. Second, I've lost my arrogance, but kept my confidence (Lesson Five: It can happen to me, and I can survive). I've accepted that I am indeed a mortal and no longer bulletproof. So many people are walking around without a clue. They don't treat themselves well and they don't take precautions. I can now take full advantage of those precautions. I've had the warning and consequently am watching myself and have others watching and monitoring with me.

One of the most horrible feelings I know is finding out death is growing in you when you had no idea. Invasion and betrayal. Eventually your body lets you know—a lump. You may sense something is wrong, but all too many times you find out too late. I feel confident that what I've learned about breast cancer is the most powerful weapon I have against it. You can't solve a problem that you don't know is there. And once you know it's there, you can't just lie back and hope it goes away. You have to take action.

# Who Killed the Shark?

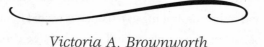

*Victoria A. Brownworth*

THIS IS A STORY ABOUT CANCER. This is a story about memory. But it is also a play, a stage production, a performance piece, because the players in the piece are performers—a performance artist, a writer—and because cancer demands many roles: patient, martyr, heretic, lunatic, stoic, heroine, villain, saint, sinner. And so at times this piece will lapse into poetics. At times it will veer into anger. At times it will take on the intonation of prayer, while at other times it may momentarily brush sentimentality. This piece will ruminate and it will castigate, but inevitably it will tell a tale: about cancer, about memory.

This piece will purport to be about one woman, but in fact will be a tale about many women. It will claim to be a piece about the first woman the author ever lived with, but it will inevitably also be about the author. It will always, even when the piece seems to be about something else, be about cancer. There will be inconsistencies. Not of fact, nor of chronology, but of elucidation. Because cancer is unclear—except when it is clear-cell cancer. Cancer is murky—except when it is the sharply delineated tumor on the x-ray film. Cancer is opaque—except when it is the bright red spot on the CT scan. So let us agree for the sake of this tale and the winding ribonucleic path it will take that cancer is never just one thing. Thus a story about cancer, particularly about one lesbian who died of cancer and another lesbian who didn't, is a story that inevitably has a Rashomon quality, a story that can be told again and again and by only changing a very few details the story can become almost any lesbian's story. It can become your story. It may already be your story.

The story—or stories, because cancer is never a singular tale and like our very DNA threads and rethreads, linking us to genetics we did not know we had—yes, the story begins in several places and times because cancer is a parallel universe to our own. It begins in Camden, New Jersey, in 1949, but it also begins in a dark lesbian bar on a chill Saturday night in Philadelphia in 1973. It may have begun at a plastics factory in New Jersey in 1968, or it may have begun at a different factory in 1971, a packing plant down the road from the plastics factory, or it may have begun with a pack of Winstons—hardpack—in a Camden schoolyard in the early sixties. The story may also have begun in utero, as a young pregnant woman smoked pack after pack of Kools as she worked on a factory assembly line, not the packing plant and not the plastics factory but in the same small New Jersey town, trying to get through one more intolerable shift.

This particular tale has an end, after four hospitalizations, three surgeries, two courses of radiation and one attempt at assisted suicide. This tale has an end, in a hospice, on a different chill Saturday night in Philadelphia.

A parallel story may have its genesis at the Jersey shore sometime in the early sixties, or perhaps in Louisiana in the late seventies. Certainly the tale does not end in an operating room in Philadelphia in the early eighties, nor in that same operating room in the mid-eighties, nor in that same operating room in the late eighties, nor in a different operating room in the early nineties, nor in a series of operating rooms throughout the nineties until the very last days of the millennium. This tale may also have its genesis in a cardboard box factory on the Delaware River in 1970, or at a gas station downwind from the oil refineries in South Philadelphia during a long, intolerably hot summer in 1971, or in one smoke-filled bar or restaurant or strip club after another throughout the seventies. This story could also have been born out of the fertile soil of the San Joaquin Valley in California during an impossibly hot summer in the last decade of the millennium. Or at a toxic waste dump upland from the Valley. Or in a field outside of Bakersfield onto which pesticides drifted like snow on a fog-filled morning in late July. Or the source of this tale may have been a pill given to a young woman sometime in the late fifties for morning sickness, a woman who smoked Newports constantly to quell her nervousness and nausea.

As historians we are taught, in college, in graduate school, to research our sources. Primary sources are best. Secondary sources are nearly as good. Tertiary sources are accepted but not preferred. As reporters we are taught, on and off the beat, in the newsroom and on the lonely, unforgiving streets, that named sources are best. Unnamed sources are accepted but not preferred. And so as the historian and reporter researching this story, I seek to know my sources, I try to get to the root, the primary point at which the tale can be said to have begun: the geneaology of the story, its genetic as well as metaphysical roots. But with cancer the leads are difficult to follow; with cancer the sources refuse to reveal themselves. With cancer sources disguise themselves or are shunted aside by other, more obvious sources: It *must* be the pack of cigarettes, not the polychlorinated biphenyls—PCBs—emitted from the liquid plastics pressing out the records sliding one after another onto a plate for eight hours at a time, leaving fumes that won't wash off for days. It must be the pack of cigarettes, not the ephemera of pesticides drifting like a perfect but implausible snow on a hot July morning, a snow that causes a slight burning in the eyes and throat and then a red prickly rash, like a childhood disease, for several days after.

Let's say it *is* the cigarettes. We've determined the source: cigarettes. But *whose* cigarettes? The Kools smoked by the young mother in the factory, or the Winston hardpack smoked by the daughter, years later? The Newports smoked by the young pregnant mother taking the drug with the three initials, DES (diethylstibestrol), or the myriad types of cigarettes smoked by the customers in the bars, restaurants and strip clubs where the daughter worked for more than a decade?

You see, cancer is an insidious story to follow.

As a child fascinated with science and medicine, I read biography after biography about famous scientists and doctors. By the age of ten I knew more about diseases of the tropics—malaria, yaws, yellow fever, Dengue fever—than most adults would ever know. I had learned about the special scourges visited on the inner city—typhoid, tuberculosis, cholera, bubonic plague. From Albert Schweitzer to Elizabeth Blackwell, from the jungles of the Congo to the slums of New York City, I knew what these scientists, these doctors battled and where.

I could explicate complicated scientific theories, albeit in the language of a child. I knew who discovered the cures for this, that, the other, and how they were discovered—Louis Pasteur, William Jenner, Robert Semmelweiss. I knew them all as well as the genesis of their discoveries, the cures that would save hundreds of thousands of lives. I knew about anthrax and how it was disseminated thirty years before it became the terroristic threat of the nineties. I knew that the Curies, Marie and Pierre, were eventually killed by the very element—radium—they had discovered.

When I was a child, cancer was the mystery illness that no one discussed. "The Big C," my parents called it. As with certain other mystery illnesses of the past, most notably tuberculosis and typhoid, classism had, inexplicably but inextricably, become attached to cancer. Cancer was a disease of the lower classes. Nice people didn't die from cancer. In the biographies I read as a child, for example, the middle-class Curies suffered from the scientific-sounding "radiation poisoning," not the cancer they developed from working with radium for two decades.

And so as I learned about one disease after another, one scientific process after another, the genesis of each disease, the process of each discovery was revealed to me. But the lesson I learned about cancer was ignorance.

This is how we resist cancer: by denying its sources.

And so as I attempt to uncover the primary sources for this story I am presented with bits and pieces of interlocking histories that may or may not add up to a sum of scientific evidence, even though all of the pieces are factual.

Some facts are immutable. *The macrosettings:* East Coast America, South

Jersey and Philadelphia, predominately, with brief forays into the Deep South and central California. Interestingly from a statistical and observational perspective, the cancer vector of the United States. *The microsettings:* fume-ridden factories and smoke-filled bars, pesticide-laden fields and chemical-laced water, shore resorts and swamplands saturated with and steeped in DDT.

Other facts are equally definitive.

Sharyn La Bance was born into a working-class family in Camden, New Jersey, in November 1949. By 1967, when she graduated from high school, she was a butch dyke who hung out in queer bars across the Delaware River in Philadelphia. She had dreams of moving to Greenwich Village and becoming an artist. Instead, she became another Camden factory worker, moving from plant to plant. One day Sharyn's hand got caught in some machinery; an index finger was severed in the accident. The missing digit became part of her butch bravado, along with the pack of cigarettes she always had rolled in the sleeve of her T-shirt.

I was eighteen when I met Sharyn at Rusty's, a one-room dive of a dyke bar on a tiny side street in Philadelphia's red-light district. Lanky and tough, in tight black jeans and a blue work shirt, with slicked back hair cut in a DA in the back, Sharyn was the prototypical butch of that era. She was tough and her friends were tougher; each had knives and knew how to use them; each could turn a beer bottle into a weapon in an instant. While I worked as an activist in the budding gay liberation movement, where violence was verboten and androgyny was queen, Sharyn and her friends swung their beer bottles and their fists in the bars where butch and femme strictly delineated every woman who passed through the door.

Less than a year after meeting Sharyn, whom I would later name Shark, from Kurt Weil's *Three Penny Opera* ballad "Mack the Knife," I had moved out of my parents' house and into an apartment with her in Philadelphia. The relationship lasted about eighteen months, until I met someone else and moved out. But Sharyn kept the name Shark and we stayed in touch over the years, although we were never close again—until the end.

*The end.* That would be the end of her life. Shark died ten days after her fiftieth birthday. The last time I saw her, she had come to my house with our mutual friend, Roberta, who cared for Shark the last two years of her life. Shark's hair, typically dyed jet black and cut in a severe straight page boy, had gone totally grey at the temples; she seemed too exhausted to dye it black. Her skin was leathery and had a gray-green tinge to it, like the sky before a tornado, an unnatural color I associate with dying.

She was anorexically thin, weighing about a hundred pounds on a frame used to carrying forty pounds more. Her black jeans hung from the backs of her legs, and her gray T-shirt seemed huge on her wraithlike body. It was midsummer and the heat was paralyzing for me. I didn't really want to have this death-visit, but intractable pain had made Shark decide she would kill herself in the coming week. The plans had been made, and she was saying her good-byes. Throughout the visit Shark paced back and forth across my living room; the pain medication made her alternately sleepy and agitated. Sitting was too uncomfortable because of a tumor pressing on the base of her spine.

I told stories; this is what storytellers do, and this was part of her reason for visiting: to be reminded of our collective past. I regaled Shark and Roberta and my lover, Judith, with tales of our misspent youth: bar fights and driving on back roads in New Jersey with the lights off and getting stoned watching Julia Child on PBS in the afternoon in the Camden apartment Shark shared with my then–best friend, Pat, who had died of liver cancer four years earlier.

The historian and archivist of the group, I brought out photographs of years past. There we are: Shark in a leather jacket, black jeans and lace-up leather boots, hair slicked back, a fake tattoo on her neck, ubiquitous cigarette in her hand; I in black leotard and tights, a long flowered skirt and platform shoes with pale blonde hair cascading over my shoulders. The photo is black and white, but I remember that the chiffon scarf tied around my neck was turquiose. Shark has her arm around me; I have my hip thrust out seductively. It is a classic photo of a classic butch-femme couple, by a lesbian photographer we both knew. The photograph had been the invitation for a show of the photographer's work. Shark is twenty-six, I am nineteen.

*See us, how young and healthy we look?*

Shark begins to cry. *It doesn't seem that long ago,* she says. It is the old cliché: *It seems like only yesterday.* And I agree. There are other photos: Christmas at my parents', my twenty-first birthday party, a gay pride event. We're hammered in all of them; it gives us a kind of naive look, the drunkenness; we seem bemused. If we had known then that we had so little time, would we have stayed sober all the time or would we have drunk ourselves into oblivion?

I do not ask this question.

Instead, I ask the question I always ask everyone: *So—what are you working on?* I say this not to be cruel but to be kind, as I know Shark has been working on some kind of memoir performance piece. She knows she won't be giving it herself, but I think she thinks somehow it will get done. Perhaps by one of us, perhaps not. She has already made plans for her memorial service. She asks me to do a eulogy and I say yes, even though I have long ago stopped going to funerals and memorial services because that is how I choose to remove myself from the epidemics—cancer and AIDS—that have defined my entire adult life. I only go to the funerals of old people now.

I do not tell her this.

As it turns out, I *will* eulogize her, although someone else will read the eulogy, not me, because the gay/lesbian/bisexual/transgendered but not disabled-accessible center in our town does not allow me access to her service after all. But the eulogy tells a story about Shark's life and her name and her history, and Roberta, Judith and others tell me later that people laughed and cried. That is what Shark would have wanted, so it is enough.

After we discuss the memorial service, we talk about the party afterward. Now would be the time to get up for a snack or go to the loo if you tend toward squeamishness. This is the part of the story where some people cover their eyes and ask another in the audience to tell them when it is all right to look. There will be other points in the story like this; this is just the first.

Shark will be cremated, and she wants a party after her memorial service at the Bike Stop, a leather bar on a tiny side street in what used to be Philadelphia's red-light district but is now the theater district; thus the setting is apropos. This bar is actually two doors up from the bar in which Shark and I met twenty-five years earlier, but I do not mention this. Instead, I listen as she blocks out the stage directions for her last performance, her postdeath scene.

*Setting:* The Bike Stop bar in high summer. The bar has French doors on the first and second floors. These windows are always open in the summer, and the cobblestoned street below, just barely wide enough for a small car to pass through, is always filled with people milling about from the bars. Shark wants us to scatter her ashes out of the second-floor window of the bar, onto the street—and the passersby—below.

*Collective gasp from the audience in my living room.*

My lover, who has always had a keen sense of the macabre, finds the idea hilarious, a perfect performance piece, and readily agrees to participate. Roberta, whose parents were both cremated and whose remains reside in little shrines along the stairwell of her tiny house, reminds Shark that there are pieces of bone that are not incinerated in the cremation. Remains are not, I remind her, like in the movies, where they are literal ashes, a fine dust blowing gently in a breeze out to sea (for that is where people always want their ashes scattered, out to sea).

I then recount the tale of my grandmother's burial. My grandmother's remains are delivered in what can only be described as a bakery box, because my mother's religious beliefs demand the "body" return to the earth as soon as possible, so there is no urn, no inviolable container. This flimsy cardboard will biodegrade quickly. None of us has ever seen cremated remains sans urn before. We expect the classic movie scene and are unprepared for the jaded cemetery attendant who arrives late, a cigarette hanging from the side of his mouth, strides up to the hole dug for the container and tosses the box into the hole like someone tossing a stone into a lake. We hear a sound like cookies shaken in a cake box. It is utterly macabre and the graveside mourners are aghast.

I suggest to Shark that most people would be repelled to find human remains hitting them on the head on a summer's evening as they cruised the street outside the Bike Stop. Shark makes the point that this is what her performance piece is all about. We discuss this at length but remain undecided about what will be done. We discuss the legalities and the logistics; it's illegal to disseminate human remains in the city limits. My perspective is that of the unwitting players on the street; the prospect strikes me as grisly. I imagine myself washing constantly and never being able to get the dust of death off me. My lover, conversely, has become quite taken with the performance idea, more than willing to participate in Shark's final staging.

I do not say what I think about death, in performance or otherwise. We change the subject.

This will be our last visit.

But I have jumped ahead of the story, as I said I might. Let me go back to the beginning. Or one of the beginnings.

The relationship ends. I move in with another woman; Shark moves into a dyke collective. I finish college, leave Philadelphia, join the domestic Peace Corps and become a journalist instead of a doctor. Shark gets involved with a series of artists and begins her own career as a performance artist; although she never goes to Greenwich Village, she gets good reviews in Philadelphia. Shark gives up factory work and cleans houses for a living.

At this point in the tale, the play or the performance, someone comes onstage and holds up a card which reads: *Twenty years pass.*

In those two decades Shark becomes well known in the Philadelphia arts community, and I become well known as a journalist, writer and activist. Occasionally our paths cross, mostly at the health food store we both frequent. We talk in the produce aisle or beside the teas or in the back where they make the fresh tofu dishes. Sometimes we stand outside so she can have a cigarette while I sit in my car. Sometimes she is with a lover, sometimes I am with mine. We talk about books mostly, or something of mine she has read, or a political point she wants to debate with me.

Sometimes we see each other at galleries. It is here I am reminded of how much closer we have come to be in later years than we were when we were younger. Sometimes I think the best thing that happened to her was she met me and moved to Philadelphia. I never say this, but when she is dying, she tells me this and I am pleased. As young as she is dying in Philadelphia, I am sure she would have died far younger in Camden.

Here, then, is the point in the play where someone steps to the front of the stage and speaks directly to the audience: "You see," this person says. I say "person" because invariably this role is played by a man, so I see a man in my mind's eye, but in fact I think it should be a woman because I am gynocentric. Perhaps it is a passing woman, or a transgendered woman, which would be fitting, as in Shark's later years she hung out with a largely transgendered crowd and she herself had been a passing woman on and off. So this passing woman steps to the edge of the stage and says, "You see, Shark was poor all her life. She never had money, she never had privilege. She had a high-school education and it wasn't a good one. She never read much of anything until she met Victoria. Her circumstances, because that's what women have always had, since time immemorial, *circumstances*, were marginal. In another time Shark might have been a character in an Edith Wharton novel—the woman who inevitably dies from lack of prospects. Or a character in George Eliot, drowning in the Floss or some other tributary of poverty and lack of privilege. Probably Eliot, because Victoria has always loved *Middlemarch* and forces all her lovers to read it.

"And," the woman continues, "cancer was there all the time anyway, so it was all much more serendipitous than anyone ever thought. Because all the while that Victoria and Shark thought there was, as Andrew Marvell wrote in 'To His Coy Mistress,' 'world enough and time,' the big clock was ticking out. That doomsday clock we all have, not just the planet, although that one is getting close to midnight, and everyone has forgotten Rachel Carson and her admonitions about the 'silent spring.' The winters have gotten drier and the summers hotter and the ice caps are melting. Did you hear about the glacial sheer the size of Rhode Island? Or that the oceans are filling with the meltoff and the coastlines are going under water—only a few inches now, but that few inches has already had a terrible impact on croplands and fishing villages and little hamlets dependent on a coastline that doesn't vary? A lot of those places are under water now, flooding every time there is even a small storm and so for those little villages the big clock has already ticked out. Tick, tick, tick.

"You see," says the woman, and now I see her more clearly. She is small and compact and dressed as one might dress a modern-day Puck if one were staging a queer version of *A Midsummer Night's Dream*. She has a boyish look, like she stepped out of an Alison Bechdel cartoon or a yeshiva. In fact, now I see that she looks like my lover, Judith, in her tweedy jacket and vest and tie.

*Who Killed the Shark?*

The light from the stage is yellow. Now I don't like the yellow spot, but it illuminates our Puck in a particular way that is both fetching and rather alarming. She looks just a tad cadaverous in this light, which seems right for this particular performance.

"So," she says, our Puck, "Shark was destined to die, regardless. Have we forgotten about the impact of environmental racism and classism? When was the last time you saw a chemical plant or an incinerator or a nuclear power silo in a middle-class neighborhood? This was the environment into which Shark was born, in which she grew up, in which she worked for decades. So there's some hubris attached to Victoria thinking that bringing Shark to Philadelphia—and may we remind the audience that we are talking about a girl who was only eighteen at the time and still had to use a fake ID to get into the very bar where she met the woman?— would save Shark's life or buy her time or prevent cancer from taking root when it did. Because as Victoria's mother always used to intone: *Blood will tell.* And who is to say what the genetics are that create a cancer that kills young? Certainly the owners of the plants and incinerators and toxic waste dumps and landfills believe *blood will tell*, that those born into these neighborhoods lead lives of less value than those, like themselves, who can afford to live elsewhere. A self-fulfilling prophecy, then: *Blood will tell*—because after the toxic waste has invaded and inveigled the DNA of entire clans, cancer becomes something handed down for generations, like china or silver would be in a family far away from air thick with pollutants."

After this soliloquy, Puck steps back into the darkness of the stage, the yellow spot goes out and the stage lights come up; the players themselves are reilluminated and return to action, the impending denouement and climax of the performance.

It is difficult to say how long Shark had the cancer before her diagnosis. Later she would tell me, in a long telephone conversation during one of her interminable hospital stays, that she had had trouble swallowing for nearly a year before she went to the clinic. She was afraid, she tells me. She didn't know who to talk to, where to go. She had no money for health care.

And that is such a common story, I think as I consider what I saw in the Central Valley in California—all the children of farmworkers dying or already

dead from the contaminating pesticides, the tainted drinking water, the subdivision housing built on landfills riddled with PCBs and other toxic chemicals. The parents of these children disbelieving that where they worked or
lived, the meager provisions they had made for their children, striving for
better lives for their children, all they could afford, had been what had killed
them. Young children, toddlers, infants, newborns. Tiny coffins lining the
landscape like in those Mexican Day of the Dead shadowboxes. Except this
is real.


This is such a common story, as I remember myself in Louisiana, sick for weeks
on end with some mysterious malady I attributed to the ungodly heat. But
there was no working plumbing where I lived and we stood in a bathtub slick
with slime day after day and drank water that exuded an odor of mothballs.
Later I heard that all the camphor trees had died the year before from some
blight and had ended up in the water supply, which the EPA had labeled the
second worst water supply in the nation. I remember sitting, sweating with
fever and shaking with delerium, in a ward in Charity Hospital only to be
told, *no money, no treatment* because that was back when such things were
totally legal.

*No money, no treatment.*

All these disparate threads weave through the story. The story that is
cancer.

Now the tale turns very, very grisly. It will churn your stomach, it will
make you wish to avert your eyes. But you should look. Look hard. This could
be someone you know. This could be you.

The pain in her gut led Shark to the clinic. The pain and a flu-like thing
that had lasted for several weeks, making it impossible for her to work. She
was out of money and needed to work. But she was in too much pain to do
much of anything. She couldn't work. So she went to the clinic, a butch dyke
whose stoicism had kept her from doctors much of her life, a butch dyke with
no money, a butch dyke fearful of what was wrong.

Here the stage directions call for a woman who looks what Radclyffe Hall
would call "mannish." The clinic sees a woman nearing fifty in tight black

jeans and a black T-shirt and black hair dyed to match. The clinic sees a woman with a short temper made shorter by pain. The clinic sees a poor woman, a mannish woman, a woman nearing fifty, with a transgendered male friend and a bad attitude.

The clinic does not examine Shark thoroughly. The clinic presses on an abdomen that is protuberant as a pregnant woman's. The clinic presses on an abdomen so tender and guarded that the woman whose abdomen it is screams involuntarily, which is something butch women never, ever do.

Yet despite these facts, the clinic proffers a diagnosis of stomach virus and acid reflux and advises over-the-counter medications for symptomatic relief of same. The clinic also advises an enema for constipation, a symptom rarely related to stomach virus or acid reflux.

Shark goes home and takes an enema. The subsequent pain is so extraordinary she passes out.

That is because her intestines have just ruptured. Because Shark does not have stomach flu or acid reflux; she has stage-four colon cancer.

In the play, the character should be dead now, not merely unconscious. But in this performance she is not dead; rather she weaves in and out of consciousness for a day or so and then calls a friend to take her to the emergency room.

There she is cursorily examined. She is treated rather roughly, as if she were one of those people who goes from emergency room to emergency room seeking pain medication for an illness that is really addiction. She is ranting a bit; she has a very high fever and is in tremendous pain. She is treated as someone marginal, what the psych wards call "borderline." She is not borderline, although that is no crime; rather, she is dying.

No blood is drawn, which would show the extraordinarily high white blood cell count because of the deadly peritonitis or the low red cell count from blood loss due to internal injury. The vital signs that indicate severe dehydration are missed or ignored. The high fever is missed or ignored. The distended abdomen is also missed or ignored. The extremity of pain is ignored. The patient is ignored.

Shark is sent home with an admonition to rest and drink plenty of fluids.

She returns to her third-floor walk-up apartment, where she spends the night in pain so intolerable that she cannot sleep. In the morning she calls another friend and asks to be returned to the emergency room.

This time the severity of Shark's physical state—she is in extremely critical condition—cannot be ignored. This time the friend who takes her to the hospital demands care for her. It is determined that she has had some sort of internal rupture and has lost much of her bodily fluids. The doctors are unable to find a vein in which to insert an IV for fluids. They put in a central line, which is inserted into the jugular vein in her neck. In doing so, the doctors puncture her lung.

Shark is taken to surgery where hundreds of gallons of distilled water are used to flush the putrefaction from her gut, which is filled with three-day-old excrement and rotting tissue. And cancer. Lots and lots of cancer, which is now out of the discrete container of her intestines and has sloshed all over her internal organs. The spores of cancer have touched all of her.

The surgeons remove Shark's colon and give her a colostomy. They note a huge tumor near her uterus but are unable to access it from the front and, because she is now slit open like a gutted fish, she cannot be turned over and cut open from behind as well. They sew her up and hope for the best. For now she is alive.


This is the end of act two. For those conversant with tragedy and opera, death always follows serious illness in the final scene. The lights dim as Shark is wheeled into recovery. Her status is critical but stable.

Puck returns in the interim to make some commentary on our tale. Since she is Judith, as well as Puck, she carries the head of Holofernes this time. Holofernes, in this case, being metaphorical. Holofernes representing the medical establishment which has just, nearly, practically, killed Shark. And so it is the role of Judith a/k/a Puck to hold high the head of Holofernes as testament to the slaughter of the innocents: here, those with cancer.

Puck reminds the audience that Shark has no medical insurance, and that this fact will play a central role in the final act of the drama. She also reminds the audience of a few statistics as well. Holofernes's head has been exchanged for pie charts and graphs. Puck notes that the uninsured poor are less than half as likely to survive any major surgery as those with insurance. She also notes that cancer kills more quickly in those without insurance or the means for what is termed "stress-free" care because the poor with cancer are inevitably diagnosed later, receive inadequate care and have no resources to provide for an extended convalescence. Puck notes that the single most common cause of homelessness—after addiction—is illness. She points to a chart that indicates that colon cancer is the third leading cause of cancer deaths in women, following lung and breast cancer. Few survive stage-four colon cancer, which nearly always metastasizes.

Puck shakes her head slowly, dramatically.

Now Puck alerts the audience to some footnotes to the story. One is that Shark's mother died of cancer five years before Shark has her surgery. Lung cancer that metastacized to her brain. An ugly death, as if any death can be said to be pretty. A painful, drawn-out death that may have begun with a pack of menthol cigarettes in the forties or may have been traveling down the assembly line at the factory where she worked or may simply have been wafted through the air from the chemical plants in the New Jersey cancer vector in which she lived.

Puck reminds us that Shark watched her mother die and this image—this series of images—haunts her. She has long said that she will not die this kind of death herself; she will choose a different exit, one predetermined by herself, rather than by her genetic material or by a rampant cell.

Shark tells me this when we talk, as she is recovering from the surgery. She wants to die now, from the pain and from the mortification of the colostomy. I tell her it will be better in a few days, a week, two weeks, that abdominal surgery is the most painful there is and that incrementally she will feel better. More than anything Shark hates the colostomy bag. The fit isn't right and she doesn't think she can ever get used to it. I tell her stupid jokes my surgeon told me, that the worst thing about a colostomy is finding shoes to match the bag. She laughs, weakly, but I know there's no humor in it. She wants to die, she tells me again. *Now.*

The morphine has made her a little buggy; at night she has hallucinations of people running in and out of her closet and bathroom. She can't sleep well; her dreams are riddled with death and bad omens. The nurses are curt; they don't really understand Shark, and she isn't good at being polite. Her friends come to visit—men dressed as women, women dressed as men, a lover of indeterminate gender and someone else who refers to himself as Shark's slave. The nurses are uncomfortable and avoid her. The doctors are uncomfortable because they have nearly killed her and now must face their mistake. No one wants to tell her the truth: that she is dying.

My own doctor, a doctor I no longer see, had seen her once and also felt uncomfortable with her butchness. I call this doctor and ask her about lawsuits, about malpractice.

*I want someone to blame.* The hospital, the doctors, the clinic seem likely candidates. I never consider the pack of cigarettes, the packing plant, the plastics factory, the genetics of parents or water or air or *circumstance*.

But this doctor, a doctor whom I will later realize has also misdiagnosed me, closes ranks, yells at me, asks why I don't just get a burial plot for Shark. She slams the phone down after telling me I am being negative, that there is always hope.

"False hope," notes Puck, coming to the front of the stage, "is either a redundancy or a catachresis. The very nature of hope is that it is false, untrue, contrary to what *is*. Conversely, hope is what allows us to continue in the face of impending doom, the sure knowledge that we will, one way or another, die. Some of us will die sooner, some of us will die later. Some of us will die smooth easy deaths, and others will linger, suffering beyond all reason. Hope, false or otherwise, is what propels us forward in the face of such knowledge. Hope is what keeps us from being paralyzed constantly by the abject terror of knowing the truth."

Puck continues: "In the creative visualization demanded of us in the new millennium, hope is what motivates us to continue living in the face of death. The quixotic element, however, is that hope is really denial, which is one of the five stages of death depicted by Dr. Elisabeth Kübler-Ross in her definitive work on coming to terms with dying. And so the dying person finds herself trapped in a schizophrenic dichotomy: She is told, repeatedly, that she must never give up hope. But she is also admonished that she must not be in denial.

"But *they are the same thing*. Hoping to survive against insurmountable odds is considered brave by some—the same people who think you are crazy if you believe you will win the lottery."

Shark did not win the lottery. She left the hospital, recovered a little, returned once to have the colostomy permanently adjusted and was told by the oncologist that she was "cancer-free," that she didn't need chemotherapy. The tumor near her uterus was determined to be something to "watch" rather than remove, the pain it caused considered "irrelevant" to the final outcome of her case.

Shark recovered, but not enough to work, so Roberta supported her. Other friends, most of them as poor as Shark, helped a little. Roberta, a social worker for more than thirty years, fought with hospitals and social service agencies and Medicare. Shark had to prove she had worked to get Social Security disability benefits. But much of what she had made cleaning houses had been paid to her in cash. And so, sick as she was, she had to call those for whom she had cleaned, many of whom had sent her money while she was recovering, and ask for letters stating that she had worked for them, that they had paid her illegally.

This is not what is meant by stress-free care.

After the second surgery Shark remained in a holding pattern for a few months and then got sick again, being admitted for surgery when she presented at the emergency room with an intestinal blockage. She spent a couple of weeks in the hospital, had the blockage—caused by adhesions and scar tissue from the previous two surgeries—removed. During this operation it was determined that the tumor growing between her uterus and spine was inoperable, but it might respond to radiation. Weak and wrung out, Shark was sent home on Christmas Eve 1998, to her third-floor walk-up apartment without a nurse or a friend to stay with her; without anyone to make her a meal or help her bathe or irrigate her colostomy bag, which had been reattached that morning. Roberta waited at the pharmacy for three hours to get Shark's medication. She left a message later that night, checking on Shark who never answers her phone, who only ever checks her voicemail messages.

On Christmas Day Shark collapses on the floor of her apartment. She has been sent home with an improperly reconnected colostomy; all her bodily fluids are leaking out of her onto the floor of her apartment, although she does not realize that this is what is happening to her. Once again, she is near death.

"One thing no one understands about butch dykes, except perhaps other butch dykes," Puck steps forward to explain to the audience, "is that we are used to being the ones to provide help. We are discomfited by asking for help. In fact, we don't really understand *how* to ask for help. And as a consequence we often find ourselves in trouble. Sometimes in a back alley with a bunch of guys who tried to get wise with us. Sometimes on the floor of our own apartment, our very life leaking out onto the carpet, and not knowing how, or whom, to call for help."

As we said, it is Christmas Day and everyone who has a family is with them. Roberta is out in rural Pennsylvania with her brothers and their wives and children. Shark's other friends are also out of town. Shark calls Roberta and leaves a message. She calls another gay male friend who tells her he will call 911.

But when the ambulance arrives, the attendants are surly and unforgiving. Shark calls to them from the window that she is too weak to climb down the stairs on her own. They tell her she either walks down or they leave, her choice. When she staggers to the street, they don't even help her into the ambulance—she must climb up the steps on her own.

Once again she is in critical condition. Once again the cause is inadequate care due to her lack of insurance, her poverty, her butch dyke persona, her marginal place in the world.

"An axiom of the AIDS epidemic," Puck reminds us, "is 'the virus does not discriminate.' We might borrow that phrase and say that cancer does not discriminate, although that may not be exactly true, because as we told you earlier, there is environmental classism, environmental racism, environmental sexism. Cancer is, first and foremost, a 'lifestyle' disease—a disease caused by how and where you live. The poor get bombarded with toxins. The poor are urged to smoke. The poor can't afford organic vegetables and fresh fruits out of season. The poor eat nitrates and smoke to mitigate the stress of their daily lives. So cancer, unlike AIDS, *does* discriminate."

Puck retreats, then returns to add this: "But nothing discriminates like privilege, and Shark didn't have any. She also didn't have insurance coverage. Poverty discriminates. They can't say anymore, as they did when Victoria staggered into Charity Hospital with a fever of 104, chills and some strange rash: *No money, no treatment.* That's not legal in the new millennium. But they can send you home on Christmas Eve without nursing care; they can send you home because there is no money for your care and you are doing damage to the hospital's bottom line."

Puck turns her back to the audience and says from under the cadaverous yellow spotlight, in a voice that seems to come from the other side, "They can send you home to die so you don't clutter their mortality and morbidity report with unwanted statistics like a poor butch dyke performance artist with fringe friends dead from delayed diagnosis followed by one botched treatment after another."

Puck turns her fine-boned head with the hair close cropped like a chemotherapy patient's and says over her shoulder, *"Out of sight, out of mind. Blood will tell."*

What surprised everyone who knew Shark was that she didn't die. Everyone knew this was the end of the third act, but she was still alive. The surgeons and oncologists told her different things at different times. They told her chemotherapy would give her another four to six months, they told her it would be mild, she wouldn't lose her hair, she wouldn't be nauseous.

I knew they were lying.

They suggested a round or two of radiation to shrink the tumor pressing against her spine. It wouldn't hurt, it would give her time, it would be benign (unlike her cancer), they told her. Just a few minutes every day for a few weeks. All she'd feel was a little sunburned at the site.

I knew they were lying.

She looked at her hand—no straight, no flush—weighed the odds, chose the radiation. It exhausted her, and didn't shrink the tumor. She decided it was time to die. She couldn't face another hospitalization or any more surgery, and the cancer and adhesions would continue to create new blockages in what remained of her digestive tract. The next trip to the hospital would, her surgeon told her, probably result in her on machines that could not be disconnected until she died.

She asked Roberta for help. She asked me for help. She asked my lover for help. She bought the book *Final Exit*. She asked her surgeon what he thought about suicide; he told her it seemed the right decision. He explained that another blockage would make it impossible. He explained that certain drugs described in *Final Exit* wouldn't work for Shark because they would simply detour directly into her colostomy bag. He wrote her a prescription for antinausea medication, for when the time came, so she could keep down the pills that would take her life. But he did not write a prescription for the medications that would take her life simply, easily, painlessly.

The assisted suicide scene must happen off-stage.

"What they don't explain in the how-to suicide books," Puck explains, "in the 'literature,' are the complicating factors of assisted suicide when the assistants are not medical professionals and when the prospective suicide doesn't really want to die. A woman with cancer has developed a tolerance of massive amounts of toxic drugs. A woman with cancer—even though she may have been winnowed down to a hundred pounds or less—has the constitution of an elephant when it comes to medications. It will take more than a couple handfuls of pills and a plastic bag to bring her down.

"Then there is the power of mind-over-matter that defies all logic or physical probability. Hence the hundred-pound mother who lifts a car off her trapped child. When your head really doesn't want to die, your body, no matter how exhausted, how riddled with cancer, will fight all efforts to kill it. And that's what happened with Shark. Despite the well-planned attempt—despite her determination that she did not want to experience another hospitalization, did not want to end up hooked to machines pumping a shadow life in and out of her at regular intervals, she did not die."

The pseudodeath scene is macabre and leaves the participants—of whom I am not one—emotionally eviscerated. This is another point at which the audience may wish to leave, although I believe they should stay, riveted by the grim scene and all it metaphorizes about cancer.


I have proclaimed my aversion to—actually moral conviction against—assisted suicide during our visit, the visit during which Shark and I have tripped down memory lane together, the visit in which Shark has declared her intention to die within two weeks. The visit during which Shark, when I say perhaps she doesn't want to do this, isn't ready to let go (I do not go so far as to say what I have heard too many times myself, "They are finding new treatments every day," because I know it is too late for this), Shark says to me, her tone angry, "You aren't suggesting I stay alive, are you?" She paces back and forth across my living room, stiff with pain, her skin no longer living skin but death skin, and turns to us—Roberta, Judith and me—and says, starting to cry, "The terrible thing is, I don't want to die. I want to live so bad." She does not say that assisted suicide has become the only small bit of control she can take at this point in her fragile, pain-wracked life. But this is what she means.

And so during that visit and after, Shark asks for help planning her death. She asks me for medications that she knows I have and she also knows will kill her. She asks Roberta and another friend to be the facilitators, the assistants, those who will guide her death ship toward Valhalla. She picks a date, sets a time, has everything ready. She has said her good-byes. This is it.


*Final Exit* details the medications and the methods. The prospective suicide mixes the pills into small quantities of food over a short period of time. Not too much at once, so as not to vomit up the death elixir. Of course Shark can only eat very small amounts of food anyway, because of the cancer and the colostomy and the tumors.

*Final Exit* stipulates that after the prospective suicide falls asleep, soon to become comatose, the assistants must place a plastic bag over her head and tie it tight around her neck so that the breathing will become more and more shallow and then suffocation will occur if the pills don't kill first. But Shark has taken enough pills to kill several people several times. The bag seems redundant.

The two assistants, whom we will not name, sit at Shark's side and stroke her arms and pray for her and ask the Goddess to guide her into the light. This scene does not replicate the movies: hours pass and nothing happens. This is the anticlimax to the performance. Shark lies breathing shallow breaths, the plastic bag firmly over her head. The assistants are exhausted and drained. Horror bleeds in and out of the room as day turns to night turns to day again.

Fifteen hours pass. Suddenly Shark sits bolt upright and says, "Get this bag off my head."

Despite the pills, the bag, the desire to take charge of her own death, she remains alive. Her will to live has superseded her will to die. Shark is disappointed but also seems relieved.

*Three months pass.*

In the time between her attempted death and her actual death, Shark is in and out of hospice care. The rest of the time she lives with a good friend, a gay man who is also a nurse. But as she gets sicker and closer to death, the cancer seems to have spread to her brain. Dementia and heavy doses of morphine leave Shark disoriented and dangerous. In a disoriented state she empties the contents of her colostomy bag over her head. She accidentally sets several fires in her friend's house. She can no longer be left alone.

Roberta divides her time between running her social service agency and finding help for Shark. Hospice care is too expensive and the state won't pay for it. Roberta wants to know why, because the hospice workers are compassionate and kind and know how to care for the dying and the state-run nursing homes are the antithesis of that. Roberta finally secures a placement for Shark in a nursing home, but it is located far outside the city and Shark's friends can't get out to see her. Roberta makes the forty-minute drive twice a day, for two reasons: She doesn't want Shark to die alone, and the nursing home staff doesn't like dealing with Shark's colostomy bag. If Roberta doesn't go twice a day, the bag does not get changed and Shark might die alone.

On a Saturday night in early November, Roberta comes to visit me but is agitated and wants to leave almost immediately, even though I am ill and need her to stay and help me. She wants to go see Shark, who has been going in and out of consciousness for several days now. In these days when I am so ill myself, Shark and I are often vying for Roberta's care. An untenable situation, one that makes us all feel guilty.

Roberta leaves. Two hours later she calls me, crying. Shark died a half hour after Roberta arrived.


This closes the final act of our performance. The Shark's deathbed stands in stark relief in the center of the stage, her body a mere shadow at her death—eighty pounds on her five-foot-six-inch frame. As the lights dim over the deathbed, Puck returns with an epilogue and a query for the audience.

"Shark's cremains were never scattered out of the Bike Stop windows," she reports. "Shark died in winter, not in summer as she had planned. And no one wanted to be the person to toss her cremains onto the street and passersby below, anyway. Roberta made little coffins and split the cremains several ways among Shark's closest friends. She has a little altar in her house, like those for her parents, now for the Shark. Roberta had asked Shark to contact her when she got to the other side. In dreams Shark has come to Roberta: She is okay now, there is no more pain.

"Now this isn't one of those mystery dinner theaters," Puck asserts, a slightly jocular tone to her voice. "You aren't expected to guess whodunit. But the title of this piece is a question: *Who killed the Shark?* That question is posed to the audience for this performance, the lesbians—butch, femme, androgynous— and the nonlesbians—queer, straight, transgendered."

The spotlight on Puck shifts from the cadaverous yellow to a rich, deep red. She dons a leather jacket and black beret like the ones Shark always wore, adds a pair of dark glasses like the Shark's. She now looks like the Shark— the Shark bathed in a blood-red glow. The murdered, eviscerated Shark.

"Roberta, the one person who had always taken care of Shark when she was alive, the person who truly kept her alive for much longer than anyone expected, the person who saved her from dying homeless and alone, organized a memorial service," Puck continues. "She put together little death testaments with art Shark had drawn, liner notes from performance pieces she had given and photos of the Shark in her heyday. These little books were very nice. Shark would have liked them a lot. Roberta also arranged to have Victoria write obituaries for the local papers. She called all of Shark's friends. Victoria wrote a eulogy that told stories of the Shark's life. Some of the mourners also told Shark tales.

"But," Puck tells the audience, "like everything else in this performance, it did not happen like the movies. No synchrony of tears, no synergy of mourning. The memorial service was frought with conflict. Very few of the mourners seemed genuinely upset. The fact is," Puck says, and the red glow deepens over her, "when Shark first got really sick, a lot of her friends simply wrote her off. That happens when women get cancer, especially when they have no money, need lots of help and everyone knows they are going to die. People who never visited her, never called her, never helped her when she was sick were at the memorial service. A tad hypocritical."

Puck steps forward and removes the leather jacket. She holds it up so that in the red light it looks like a skin newly flayed from an animal. "They fought over this, you know," Puck says of the mourners and the jacket. "A group of her friends stood together at the memorial service fighting over who would get the jacket. They were touching it, fondling, cuddling it. It wouldn't have fit the people fighting over it. But there they were, supposed to be mourning Shark or at least celebrating her life. Instead, they were fighting over her only real possession: her leather jacket. They were giving that jacket the attention they never gave Shark when she was dying.

"Of course, there had already been other fights," adds Puck, slowly putting the jacket back on, taking the dark glasses off and sliding them into the jacket's inside pocket. "The man who called himself her slave, for example, who had never come to visit, had gone to the funeral home and demanded the body. Later he called Roberta and threatened to sue her for Shark's ashes. Meanwhile, the transgendered MTF who had been Shark's last lover, who had left her when she got really ill, was at the memorial service trying to pick *me* up," says Puck, repositioning herself within the leather jacket as if to reassert herself, to reestablish herself within this leather skin.

"So that was the *true* final performance—that skirmish over the jacket," Puck concludes, walking to the edge of the stage and sitting down, legs dangling into the black void of the orchestra pit. "Fitting, that. Just not a very kind performance. What no one said at the memorial service is that performance art spilled over into every aspect of Shark's life. Reality was a performance piece for her: She had discovered that for her, reality could be manipulated by her performance.

"That was true until she got cancer," Puck explains and stretches out on the stage. "She couldn't manipulate that, try as she did." Puck is now laid out on the edge of the stage, bathed in the deep red light. Behind her, at the middle distance of the stage, a cold blue spot slowly illumines the deathbed on which there now stands a little sign, like a sandwich board outside a cafe. It is beautifully calligraphed. It reads: *Who killed the Shark?*

"And so in closing this performance," Puck intones from her prone, corpselike position, "we return to our original question. Certainly cancer killed Shark," she asserts and pulls a little jar with a skull and crossbones from her pocket and holds it up. Inside is a length of intestine. A green biohazard symbol is projected against her as she lies along the stage. "But where did the cancer come from? Certainly the medical establishment killed Shark," Puck adds, holding up Holofernes's head over her gut. "But why? Why did so many different doctors ignore her, ignore how sick she was, until it was too late, until the cancer had washed through her body like a wave of death?

"These are the villains we know for sure," Puck tells the audience. She sits up, her face now white like a deathmask, her eyes outlined in black. "These are the simple answers to our question. Cancer killed the Shark and the doctors helped. But what does it mean that the people who are supposed to save us in fact may not care enough about whether we live or die to choose one fate over the other? What does it mean that we will never know what caused the cancer that killed Shark, because no one with the power to do something about it cares whether the cancer came from a pack of cigarettes or a puff of DDT or plate after plate of PCBs pressing out into vinyl records that we would all dance to later?"

Now music plays in the background. It is Gene Pitney's "Town without Pity," one of Shark's signature songs. Puck rises, begins to dance. The blood-red spot is replaced by a glitter ball that turns the stage into a dance floor, prisms of reflected light scattering everywhere. Girlie girls and butch women step into the background and dance slowly around Shark's deathbed on which Puck now reverently lays the leather jacket, the shades and the beret. She returns to the front of the stage and pulls a pack of numbered cards from her back pocket. She holds them up one at a time while pointing to different lesbian couples dancing. The scene is reminiscent of those dance contests that bars used to hold.

"Couple number one is cancer-free," notes Puck, flipping a card in their direction. "But couple number two is harboring a stage-two breast cancer and a basal-cell carcinoma. Couple number three has a dormant lymphoma and oh, yes," she looks down at her notes on the back of the last numbered card, "another breast cancer. Already metastasized, but still not yet diagnosed. Couple number four, clear. Couple number five, an incipient ovarian cancer—that's bad, really no way that's going to get diagnosed in time—and a stage-one colon cancer moving rapidly to stage two. Couples six, seven and eight—one of each couple will have breast cancer before the decade is out."

Gene Pitney fades out and Laura Nyro starts to sing "Gonna Take a Miracle." Four of the couples have left, the femmes in tears, the butches looking stricken, comforting their lovers. The others continue dancing, but it's formal and dirgelike now, none of the sensual passion of the first dance. Now they know, cancer is stalking them, has caught them. At the back of the stage tombstones are illumined one by one, by different colored spots. On them are names of lesbians—some famous—dead from cancer: Rachel Carson, Audre Lorde, Laura Nyro, Barbara Deming, many others we cannot read. The Shark's name is being carved into one tombstone with a penknife by one of the butch dancers.

"Our performance has ended," Puck announces, scattering the remaining cards into the audience. Some have tiny skull and crossbone signs on them or little biohazard symbols, others do not. "The Shark has been eulogized, her story told. And as we told you at the outset, this performance isn't just about the Shark. Any one of you could draw the cancer card in your next hand. Some of you may have already drawn it, you just don't know it yet, cancer being the proverbial crapshoot. Don't worry, you'll have plenty of time to agonize over every choice you ever made. The smoky bars and restaurants even if you never smoked yourself. The jobs you took. The way that toner made you itch when you changed the cartridges in the xerox machine. What about those rays from your computer or the TV when you were a kid and always sat right up close? How about all that lying out in the sun? Or the diet foods with aspartame. And don't forget the meat and eggs and butter before you went vegetarian or the fruits and vegetables steeped in pesticides once you did. Like I said, you'll have plenty of time to wonder what it was that killed you.

"What killed the Shark? Cancer. Poverty. Indifference. Environment. Lack of privilege. Sexism. Marginality. Homophobia. Ignorance. Cancer," Puck says. The music has now ended, the glitter ball lights dimmed and a tiny yellow spot the only light, like a little candle flame on the stage behind Puck's head. She turns her back to the audience, walks to the deathbed on which the leather jacket and shades and beret lie in state. She sits on the bed, puts her hand on the arm of the jacket as if on the arm of a friend.

Lights dim to black. Puck, white deathmask face aglow in the darkness, walks to the side of the stage, slowly pulls the curtain closed. As the curtains meet, she slides out from behind the thick brocade and addresses the audience a final time.

"The fact is, we know who and what killed Shark," Puck concludes quietly, her voice barely audible from the now-dark stage. "And when murder is committed, we seek justice. So the question is no longer who killed the Shark, it is this: *What will we do to avenge her death?*"

> *Exit stage left.*
> *The end.*

# A Tribute to Pat Parker

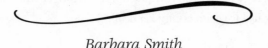

*Barbara Smith*

PAT PARKER'S POETRY IS THE FIRST explicitly Black lesbian feminist writing I remember reading. In the mid-1970s, when I came out, Black lesbians were virtually invisible both in real life and in print. *Pit Stop* and *Child of Myself* were lifelines, which provided evidence that it was not only possible to survive as a Black lesbian, but that it was possible to be an out Black lesbian writer as well.

A few years later I had the chance to meet Pat and to experience her remarkable gift for reading and interpreting her work via the spoken word. I was delighted as I got to know her that she was as down-to-earth, humorous, and caring as her writing had made her seem.

In 1978 the Black feminist Combahee River Collective, of which I was a member, helped to produce the Varied Voices of Black Women concerts in Boston during an east coast tour organized by Olivia Records. The fact that Pat—one of the four headliners with musicians Linda Tillery, Gwen Avery, and Mary Watkins—regularly brought down the house with her poetry indicates how talented she was in presenting her work to live and diverse audiences.

Audre Lorde loved Pat and deeply respected her work. Sometimes Audre mentioned when they had recently shared new writing or discussed other issues that concerned them as working poets. Audre was devastated when Pat died, especially since it was the same disease she was battling. I received untold support from Audre and Pat not only because they were sister writers, but because they were committed, radical activists who understood that a part of their work on earth was to join with others to fight oppression on many fronts, that writing was not enough.

In the early 1980s, all three of us attended a Black feminist writers conference in Eugene, Oregon. When we were going around the room discussing how we defined Black feminism and saw our work, I will never forget what Pat said. She stated that she saw herself as a revolutionary, that this was a word that people used to say all the time in the '60s and '70s, but that we did not hear much any more. She told us that what she was working for as a Black feminist and lesbian was a revolution. I vowed to myself from that day on to use the word *revolution* to define my political goals.

I miss Pat. There are more Black lesbians writing now than there were two decades ago, but there are fewer revolutionaries.

# MASSAGE
## *(for Margaret)*

*Pat Parker*

In the days following my mastectomy
my body was covered in bandages
mountains of tape hid the space
where my breast had been,
piled so high
the breast was still there.

My body was numb
hard like my mother's body
in her casket
and I mourned
mourned for the passion gone
and I numbed my mind.

No one had seen my body
except for my lover and my surgeon.

I protected my friends with robes,
my gymmates with towels

protected myself
no looks of horror
    pity
        disgust

Let the numbness be still.

I had a massage appointment
and I brought my numb self
turned my body into bread
for your hands to knead and mold
to stroke the tension
away
    away
        away

Like fine bread I rise
my body loose and smooth
    tensing
        passionate
and I want to sing

I reawake

I want to kiss you
instead I say thank you
and go home.

# It's Not So Bad

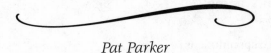

*Pat Parker*

It's not so bad
when your life is
enclosed in parentheses
    born
        died
definite and final.

It's not so bad
when the unknown
becomes known
    cause of death
        time
are projected on
scales and graphs
like tide flows.

It's not so bad
when friends ask
how are you? and
you see their bodies
    tensed
        buffered
for your answer.

It's not so bad
as the distance
    lengthens
        clear walls build
between you and
the healthy ones.

What really hurts
causes heartache
and silent screams
is to watch people
    prepare
        for your death
and you haven't.

# A Scar I Did Not
# Want to Hide

*Jerilyn Goodman*

8 A.M. SATURDAY. Less than forty-eight hours since surgery to remove my left breast. My chest is wrapped in a protective elastic bandage and two drainage tubes emerge from small incisions near my lower ribs to siphon fluid from the mastectomy site.

My surgeon, in customary manner, breezes into the room. She is going away for the weekend but has stopped in to see me, as promised. After checking the fluid levels, she announces that the tubes can come out. "Yes," I tell her, "the resident said he'll do it later in the day."

"Well, I can do it now," she offers.

I am happy to see the drains go but not prepared for what she says next. "Here's what we can do. I can take the drains out and leave the bandage on for as long as you want. Or I can take the bandage off and replace it with something smaller—you don't have to look. Or I can take it off and you can look at it."

I knew the big swatch of elastic that encircled my upper torso had been put there "for my protection"—more psychological than physical. There would be no real pain at the mastectomy site, as the nerves that had brought sensation to my breast were gone.

But I was struck dumb by the choices I had not been expecting to make. Perhaps sensing this, my surgeon plopped herself in the chair by the bed. "You don't have to look at it now. I have one patient who hasn't looked at herself in twenty years." I knew I would not be like that woman. I would be one who wanted to accept this alteration to my body with grace and pride and defiance. Single-breasted women would have to make their scars visible to demonstrate the magnitude of this epidemic. No, I would not shy away from looking at my body. But, now? Right this minute? I felt numbed by panic.

"That's what I like about you," I tried to joke in a desperate bid to buy some time. "You offer me choices so undesirable that there's only one option to choose. You know I don't want to walk around with this bandage on until I see you again in ten days." But my attempt at humor was short-lived. "What will it look like?" I asked meekly.

"It will look fine," she assured me.

"What does that mean?" I wondered, but didn't ask. Now is the time, I thought. The sooner you confront it, the sooner you can accept it. "OK," I said, "let's do it. But you look first and tell me if it's OK to look." I was forty-three, talking like a five-year-old.

She left the room and returned with a handful of supplies. We were mercifully alone, she and I—no nurses, medical students, interns, residents, loving family and friends. Just my doctor and me. As she removed the drains and snipped off the bandage, she was helping me heal through a procedure probably not mentioned in any medical text. Make the patient feel safe, make the patient feel cared for, and most important, make the patient feel in control of what is happening to her.

The road to this doctor's clinic had not been an easy one. Over the past five years, I had told an assortment of doctors about a suspicious thickening in my breast. "I don't see anything," said four different radiologists. "I don't feel anything," said three internists. "I wouldn't worry about it," said two surgeons. But I worried every day.

Things only got worse after the biopsy. I listened to the surgeon who did the needle aspiration and misled me about the results. "Atypical cells," he said, when in fact it showed cancer. He was the man who announced without discussion, "I want to do a mastectomy and I like to do reconstruction at the same time."

I persisted with the internist who, when asked if he could get me an appointment with the prominent female physician, replied, "I don't know why you need to see another surgeon." I was rejected by the oncologist who refused to make an appointment with me when told I would also be meeting with another doctor in his office.

"If you're seeing her," his assistant relayed sheepishly, "he said he doesn't need to meet you."

"But how can I choose the right doctor for me if I can't talk with him?" I asked.

"Keep the appointment with the woman and maybe he'll pop his head in and say hello."

I met with the plastic surgeon who, when I said, "I'm not sure I want reconstructive surgery," replied incredulously, "Why not!?"

After all of this, I sought out the surgeon who reviewed my records and said, "I can do a lumpectomy, here are the pros and cons. I can do a mastectomy, here are the pros and cons." I took it all in and when I asked, "Do you have a recommendation?" she offered it. She is the surgeon who at the time of my initial evaluation had me meet not only with an oncologist and a radiologist but with a psychiatrist who assessed my emotional adjustment and offered support of varying kinds. This is the surgeon who believes fervently that the more information a patient has, the better able she is to cope with her circumstances.

As the bandage fell away, I snuck glances down, waiting to be shocked by some unimaginable horror—a vision of my body, raw, wounded and bloody.

Instead, I saw clean, healthy skin and a thin band of Steri-strips covering a neat incision. It was nothing. And it was everything. I looked for what seemed like a long time and felt myself begin to breathe again.

"I'll put some gauze pads around this for your protection," she told me. "But you can take a shower tonight and these bandages can come off." As she left to go off for the weekend, we smiled proudly at each other, acknowledging our accomplishments.

That night, alone in my room, I stood in front of the bathroom mirror and took off the remaining bandages. They provided protection I didn't really need. They covered a scar I did not want to hide. They represented a level of medical care that should not be so difficult to find.

# Vigil

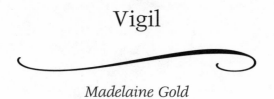

*Madelaine Gold*

*If Nora had never gotten cancer we never would have been lovers.*

I am an artist. I tell stories in images and colors and textures. But this is a story that must be told in words, even though I will never be able to articulate in language what I might say on a canvas. The tale of my relationship with Nora Alden* is one I have carried with me for over twenty years. Twenty years in which I have kept a kind of vigil—of love and memory, of loss and regret.

Most tales that begin with love and end with death are bittersweet; this story is no different. It's sad and painful and difficult to tell. But as I said, it's a story that has stayed with me for more than two decades, a story that will remain with me always, a story that should be told, and that in telling, I hope will expiate grief and remorse while also honoring my love for Nora and hers for me.

Before you can make a painting, there are preliminary steps involved. The canvas must be prepared; the fabric must be stretched tight to the frame so the paint will not slide off the canvas or warp the fabric. Then the canvas must be gessoed to temper it so that the fabric remains supple and so that the paint will adhere without drying out the canvas—this allows it to age so the painting can last for centuries. These steps form a foundation for the finished painting—without the proper preparation, the painting cannot survive.

Although we met because of art—Nora was a professor of painting in the Masters of Fine Arts program at the prestigious New York arts college where I was getting my MFA—the foundation for my relationship with her was, in many respects, her cancer. As I said, if she hadn't had cancer, we would not have become lovers. Her cancer—the possibility that she might die—gave her a kind of courage she didn't know she had before the disease. She didn't really fear dying—she feared not living her life as fully as possible. Unfortunately most of us who aren't threatened with death, who don't have a sense that our time is running out, aren't as good at taking risks. We're much more fearful of the everyday, the mundane, the ordinary. And so as Nora took risks because she had come so close to death, the rest of us—me, her family, her friends—lived caution-filled, even static lives. There are consequences to longevity that the dying do not accept.

But I am getting ahead of the story, putting the paint down before the canvas is prepared.

Classic tales of love and death have a stock cast of characters. The protagonist is a courageous hero/heroine who, we know, will die by story's end. There is a lover of the hero/heroine who doesn't quite manage to save the protagonist in the end. And of course, since the path of true love in these tragedies never runs smooth, a villain stands in the way of a happy ending. Nora's and my story followed this classic formula. Except there was more than one villain.

I was twenty-two when I met Nora; she had just turned forty. For the first two years that I knew her, she was my teacher and mentor. For the next year, which was also the last year of her life, we were lovers.

Being an artist and being a lesbian were both intrinsic for me. My parents were artists and both taught at the art college from which I received my undergraduate degree. Art—and artists—were what I had been raised with, and as a consequence I had a certain perspective on who they were. I thought most to be quite arrogant and somewhat shallow, focused solely on their own ideas, their own success and the means to that end. Nora was none of those things and at first I was disappointed by her quiet simplicity and wise nurturing of her graduate students. But as I got to know her, I grew to love her.

I had been a lesbian since high school. Nora was married to a man, had three children and had never had a female lover.

We were an unlikely match.

When I met Nora she looked older than her forty years. Her hair, once dark and lustrous, was thin from the recent chemotherapy and had turned prematurely gray. She was about five foot six, but she never really stood up straight—the pain and exhaustion kept her a little stooped. She was puffy from steroids—her face looked jowly, her skin had a sallow tinge from her illness, and her eyes, which were an incredible watery blue, were rheumy. Nora had started to look old and matronly, despite being only forty. She had been beautiful in a very traditional way when she was younger—when I went through old photographs of her, I could see the woman she would have become had she not gotten cancer. But it wasn't how she looked that attracted me to her— it was how and who she was. Nora was a very dichotomous creature when I met her— amazingly strong and incredibly fragile. Wonderfully nurturing and also self-absorbed in a way only the dying can be—she didn't care anymore what people thought. She intended to do and say whatever she wanted and was unconcerned with consequences. I felt no such luxury, mired as I was—in my youthful arrogance—in the dailiness of living.

Nora had cancer for the entire time I knew her. She was diagnosed with breast cancer at thirty-nine and underwent a mastectomy, chemotherapy and radiation. Within two years the cancer metastasized to her brain, and she died at forty-three from brain cancer.

As I said, Nora was different from anyone I'd ever met in the art world. In fact, she was the antithesis. She exhibited none of the jealousy, hostility or anger I'd come to associate with artists. She was very generous—she was willing to share her ideas and was open to new ideas. Nora wasn't arrogant, wasn't a braggart. She was warm and kind. She challenged everything I knew about the art world.

For Nora I was a challenge. I *was* arrogant. But Nora treated me more like a colleague than a student. She approached me like she was taming a wild horse. She loved my work, which was very different from hers. She was very supportive of my career and dragged me everywhere, introducing me to people, taking me to galleries. She wanted success for me. There was a lot of grooming for success for me by her—she was a mentor and then we would reach points where we were peers. There was a great deal of mutual respect.

Nora's husband, Kent, was a very handsome, charismatic womanizer in what was supposed to be an open marriage. He was a charming sleazeball, a playboy. He had used his looks and charisma to make a name for himself, but he spent more than he made and so he and Nora and their kids lived on her salary in the house the school provided for her. Tenured professors made money in those days. Her two youngest children, Emily, sixteen, and Ronald, nine, lived at home. Her oldest son, James, was twenty and already away at college when I met her.

The story of Nora's cancer and our relationship is also a story about lesbianism and what it means to different people. I said earlier that there is always a villain in a tragedy, which is what our story ultimately was. But in our story there was more than one villain—there was cancer, but there was also Kent and there was also homophobia. And as the villain in a tragedy conspires to keep the lovers apart, these three villains did just that.

After her surgery Nora viewed herself as disfigured and less womanly. She couldn't bear to look at herself, at the scars; even when she took a bath she would cover herself with a washcloth. Kent had deserted Nora emotionally and sexually after she became ill. He never touched her again after her breast surgery. He never took care of her, never went to any of her medical appointments and flaunted his affairs in her face. Kent left her care to their children and her friends. His treatment of her was another devastating event in her life.

So after the surgery and Kent's mistreatment, I think she could only be with another woman, because I think only another woman could really understand what had happened to her. I couldn't bear that she was so disturbed by how she looked, that she couldn't even look at her own body. I wanted to make her feel wanted and sexy and loved.

I told her I loved her, I told her I wanted to be with her. At first I think she was a little shocked; she had never been approached by another woman before. A week passed. Then she made up her mind: She took me away to the country for the weekend and we became lovers. I tried to show her as tenderly as possible that I loved her, that her cancer didn't matter to me, her scars didn't matter to me. I touched all those places she couldn't bear to even look at. I tried to give her back to herself, to give her a sense of herself as a woman, as a sexual being—all those things that had been taken away by the cancer and by her husband.

We grew closer and closer and the affair deepened. But her husband—despite being very profligate with other women—remained very possessive of her and very threatening. You could destroy people in those years by revealing their lesbianism. And she had her career and her children, so we were trying to figure out what we would do, how we could change our lives to make it possible for us to be together without shattering everything.

Nora was jeopardizing the personal and professional life she had built so carefully over so many years for me, but I think cancer was the catalyst. Cancer gave Nora a very different perspective on life—it imbued her with a courage and a kind of daring that she had never allowed herself before, not even in her art. Even if she had lived to be 110, she wouldn't have taken those risks pre-cancer; she was very stolid before the disease. Cancer made her conscious of the ephemeral nature of things and she was no longer willing to let passion elude her.

Nora had had wonderful and powerful relationships with women. She had strong friendships with women—her best friend was dying of stomach cancer at the same time Nora was dying of her own cancer and they were very nurturing of each other. All her deepest relationships, other than the ones with her sons, were with women. So I think it finally felt natural to her to be with another woman, to not care about what people might say, to not care if she was called a lesbian or if her marriage was destroyed. She needed the kind of love another woman could give her and she also needed very much to give love back. Kent didn't—couldn't—give her love or make her feel desired, nor did he allow her to give him love. He flaunted his profligacy in her face even when she was most ill, even as he withheld affection from her.

Our love affair was very profound for me and for Nora. I have never experienced a love that was so encompassing. Nora was a lover and a friend. She was sexy and mentoring and maternal all at once. She was the most daring lover I have ever had: She was willing to try anything new and did; she wanted to experience every possible aspect of lesbianism. With Nora, every single part of me was nurtured. I had never felt that before. It was everything to me.

I should note here that as our relationship deepened, Nora and I both thought she was getting better. She'd had the surgery; the chemotherapy and radiation were over. What we thought we were fighting at this point was the homophobia that was still quite entrenched in the late seventies. We thought the most difficult thing we had to do was try and find a way to be together without either of us losing our careers and without Nora losing her children.

We were getting closer and closer. Nora had been having headaches and flulike symptoms for about a month. One night, we were out for dinner and Nora left the table and was gone for a long time. She had a seizure in the ladies' room. I had to call Kent—who did not know the nature of our relationship—to have him pick us up. Then we all—Nora, Kent, Nora's youngest child, Ronald, and I—went down to Nora's parents' house in Virginia. There she had another massive seizure and was rushed to the hospital. She had emergency brain surgery; the surgeons removed a huge tumor that had practically caused Nora's brain to split in two. As soon as she was strong enough to travel, we all returned to New York. There Nora was admitted to the cancer hospital, Sloan-Kettering, where she remained for the months until her death.

Things had gone from bad to worse in the weeks between Nora's seizure in New York and her surgery in Virginia. While she was in Virginia her husband and her parents—born-again Christian fundamentalists—found her diary and love letters from me. Nora had told them she didn't want anyone to take care of her but me. So her parents turned the "job" of taking care of Nora over to me. When she needed something they would knock on my door and say, "Nora needs medication. Nora needs a bath." Ronald—he was only nine—helped me. Together we took care of Nora.

When we returned to New York and Nora was admitted to Sloan-Kettering for treatment, Kent made his move. He told me if I didn't have sex with him, he wouldn't allow me to see Nora. I refused and he banned me from the hospital and had her calls blocked. Nora went to the hospital not knowing why I wasn't with her. She ended up thinking I didn't love her anymore and I wasn't able to explain it to her because I didn't have any access to her.

Nora's friends resented me because I wasn't at the hospital. They thought I had deserted her because she was dying. I had told them I was her lover, but they didn't believe me because of her husband and family. Being "out" wasn't as common twenty years ago as it is now; it wasn't common knowledge that a woman could be married to a man and also lovers with another woman. I told Nora's friends that Kent was keeping me from seeing her, but again no one believed me. I didn't know what he was saying about me, but I imagined it was that I didn't care enough for my "friend" Nora to be with her when she was dying. Because Kent was Nora's husband, he had the legal power to determine who could visit her and who could not. Families still have tremendous power over what happens to their lesbian and gay family members when they are seriously ill. Parents can come in and take over; they can ban an adult child's lover from the hospital. Kent had the power to keep me from Nora and he did.

Weeks passed. I got a telephone call telling me that Nora was expected to die very soon, in a matter of days. Nora had been asking for me, asking why I wasn't there with her, and Kent had finally told her what he had done, how he had blackmailed me. Kent promised Nora he would put me on the visitor's list.

Nora called me. She told me Kent had explained everything to her. She told me she understood that I hadn't deserted her willingly. She told me she loved me. I told her I loved her. I told her I was sorry I had been kept from her. I told her I would see her the next day.

I intended to visit Nora the next day after work. But when I got home, there was a message that she had died. I was the last person to talk to her before she died. I think Nora stayed alive to talk to me. It's a horrible, arrogant thing to say, but I do believe it—that she waited for me, to talk to me, and once she had, she knew it was okay to let go and she died.

I didn't go to Nora's funeral because of her children, because of the scandal. Nora had always wanted me to take care of Emily and Ronald, but I wasn't able to. I hope one day I have the courage to contact them—I'm afraid they hate me and think I abandoned first their mother and then them, but I couldn't fight their father. Twenty years later, both of them adults, probably with families of their own, and I still don't know what I would say to them, how I would explain what happened.

It's a tragic story—the heroine dies, the lovers reunite briefly and only by telephone at the last moments before the heroine's untimely death. The villains seem to have won. But it's also a wonderful story because it is about the tremendous power of love. Nora's and my relationship changed both our lives, deepening our emotions and broadening our experience. As terrible as some parts of that time were, I wouldn't have traded one second because Nora was part of it all. The time I spent with Nora taught me more than any experience in my life. Not just about love and desire, but about what I could accept and what I couldn't, what was really important and what was insignificant. I was young—I didn't think I could deal with a lover with cancer, one breast, a shaved head. Those things became so minor. You get over it because it's the woman you love, and nothing is more important than being with her. All the things you think you know about attraction and attractiveness melt away in the passion you feel, in the desire to be together, in the fervor to keep death at bay. I was honored and privileged to be with Nora, I was fortunate to love her and fortunate to be loved by her.

I have only one regret about our time together: that I allowed myself to be blackmailed and threatened by Kent, that I allowed myself to be kept away from Nora when she was dying. For over two decades I have felt ashamed, as if I failed her.

Cancer steals so much from us—it stole Nora's breast, then half her brain, then her life. But in the midst of that assault on her body, Nora found a courage and strength she didn't know she had. She touched me with that courage; she took the risk to love me.

And so I tell our story and in the telling hope to forgive myself for how I believe I failed Nora at the end. But more important I want to tell Nora, once again, how very important she was in my life, how much I love and miss her still.

*all names are psuedonyms

# BLOOD MONEY
## August–November 1985

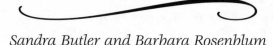

*Sandra Butler and Barbara Rosenblum*

*Sandy*

*August 6*

Barbara is nervous, preparing to give her mother and father more information about her diagnosis. They need to be prepared for the radiation, the length of time she will be on strong chemo, and still be left with a sense of optimism. A balancing act, but one that Barbara is determined to make. She sits on the window seat overlooking her garden, a yellow pad balanced on her knees, drafting all the possible directions the conversation might take.

Meeting with her cancer counselor yesterday, she was asked to describe a recent family crisis and the ways each member behaved. "That is how your family will respond this time," she was told. "Whatever their relationship to the crisis, their engagement or lack of it, their protectiveness or avoidance, it will be the same."

After she has written a likely scenario that includes their anticipated reactions, she calls me to the sofa where we rehearse the plan she has drawn up. Like a battle plan, all the pieces in place.

"What will you tell your mother when she asks why you didn't tell her everything when they were here?" I begin.

"I didn't want to worry her," she says firmly.

That is true. Barbara has never wanted to worry her parents and has kept many parts of her life from them. She has often criticized me for giving my mother what she felt was too much information. "Can't you see it will just upset her? What's the point of telling her something she can't understand and that will only aggravate her?" Good questions.

But for me the telling, however inappropriate it may have been, was always motivated by a desire to be known, to be seen by my mother. Visibility more important a consideration than protection. Barbara and I each had a relationship to "telling" that was quite different. And each equally unsuccessful.

Now, both of her parents are frail, in their mid-seventies; her mother has lymphatic cancer controlled successfully with chemotherapy, and her father is nearly blind and no longer able to work. Barbara can no longer protect them from information that will be "upsetting," "aggravating." Cancer has taken that protective option from her.

We drink tea and discuss ways to present the medical information, couch the words, make it palatable. As we plan, I find my thoughts drifting, trying to imagine receiving such a call from one of my own daughters.

How would they tell me if one of them had cancer? Would they tell each other first, as Barbara has done with her sister Ruth? My eldest daughter, Janaea, might have. She would first tell her partner, Tony, then her younger sister, Alison, and together with them face what needed to be done. She would protect me, I decide. She wouldn't want me to know until things were stable, doctors had been chosen, and treatment was already under way. Alison has no partner now, so I expect she would reach out toward me first. But if she had a partner—would she do the same? Might there be a time when I would become simply another psychological task to be managed in a time of crisis—with skill, tact, and love?

What would it feel like to know one of my daughters had cancer? What would be the "same" ways I would engage with them? What would they be able to predict from our decades together? Words, I suppose. Information, feelings, books. Talking. That's always been my answer to everything. But cancer doesn't respond to words.

I pull my attention back to what Barbara is saying. Force myself to remember the differences. Barbara's mother, Regina, barely escaped an emotionally impoverished childhood in Poland and lost nearly her entire family to the Nazis, leaving permanent scars of depression and terror at all the unforeseen dangers in the world.

David, her father, was rarely present because he worked six days a week, twelve hours a day to make a meager living for his family. Both parents, while expecting their daughters would become "workers," hoped they would go to college. They shifted all their dreams onto their children and immersed themselves relievedly in the new troubles, the little troubles, that made up their life in America.

Ruth lived too far away; Barbara had a boyfriend who was unsuitable. Barbara didn't eat well. Ruth was too thin and worked too hard. Barbara was anxious about tenure. No longer life-and-death matters as it had been for them growing up in Europe.

But now all that will change. Death and the struggle for life will enter their world again after so many decades of safety in America.

I feel disengaged and lonely as we talk. My mother, Barbara's parents, my daughters, Barbara's sister blur—a shifting series of images. The dreams I have for my children are the same as those of her parents. We share the sense of impotence at being unable to protect our children from the dangers that await them. Barbara's parents must now face the terrifying reality that their first-born may die before them. I grow fearful about losing my children. Losing Barbara. We are all in danger now.

*Barbara*

*August 7*

How do I disclose and to whom? Under what conditions does disclosure become relevant? Give it language, it becomes exposed to air. It breathes, it's alive: to tell is to make real. I must. I am impelled to reach out.

Disclosure begins as desperation, a frothing at the mouth, a constant foaming of anxiety. The anxiety is pervasive. So is my disclosure. Everyone has to know. I have no boundaries, no ability to differentiate among levels of friendship, levels of intimacy.

Later I can relax and allow enough time to elapse for me to observe and process other people's responses to me. I am able to differentiate and discriminate between friends. Some people have moved in closer. Others cannot bear to have lengthy conversations with me—they have disappeared. Others haven't visited. They haven't seen me bald or my head covered with my little cap.

Yet some, like Marinell and Stan, asked to look at my scar. Marinell even touched it.

Old lovers seem to have a harder time. T. didn't call for ten days after being told. J. has known for over a month and has not written. G. has known for at least two weeks, possibly three, and hasn't called. L. is upset and transparently ambivalent.

As I begin to observe them, I am able to classify types of response independent of previous intimacy. It's a new classification system with the heroes being "heart" people, those who can reach out, comfort, or write to share stories. People who can tolerate illness, sadness, and hardship are new friends. Those who have pulled back and not called—I don't mind. I'm not angry nor do I feel disappointed. I understand how it can be for them. Wasn't I afraid of June? Wasn't I afraid to be near her, seeing her death in front of me? Sandy is angry at them, thinking they have an obligation to overcome their own anxiety and behave with more decency. It's not that they are indecent. They are afraid.

*Barbara*
*August 10*

Today I was ecstatic, shot through with internal happiness. Even a sense of joy. Why? For the first time in a week I have energy instead of chemicals rushing through me. I can feel this energy pumping my heart and body. So much energy—three hours of intellectual energy, two hours of gardening energy. And music. Music. Singing along with Bernardo and Maria. Show tunes. Dancing with the ensemble in *A Chorus Line*. Washing that man right out of my hair.

My fingernails are dirty, chlorophyll-stained from gathering grass cuttings in the park. Four bags full for composting in my garden. Breaking up the clods, interspersing the cut grass, making the soil buoyant and light.

What extraordinary bodily pleasure to feel the stretches, tugs, and pulls in my muscles. The joy of being warm because I'm moving my body all the time. And the garden smells of earth and life. The music is loud as I shovel, dig, and get dirty. It's wonderful.

Naturally I did too much. My muscles hurt, my back aches, my shoulder is stiff from shoveling, but what pleasure! I love it—alive, alive, alive. Screaming alive. Fighting alive. Kicking alive!

*Sandy*
*August 20*

They have prepared Barbara's vulnerable chest to receive radiation, tracing a grid on it with a thick pen in geometric stains that enrage me. Pirate's treasure. "X" marks the spot. Dig it out. But her long throat and narrow shoulders seem familiar, the rest of her body remains fully fleshed and sturdy, and her hair is beginning to grow back.

This morning Barbara put on a dusty-rose blouse with puffed sleeves made of a silky fabric that rests gently upon her. Emerging from its neckline and extending towards her throat is a garish red line. Just as her relatives who survived the Nazi concentration camps had marked bodies, so I hope this too will be a mark of survival.

I look at a picture of her taken just one year ago during our holiday at Sea Ranch. She is naked, perched in front of a picture window, towel wrapped turbanlike around her head, smiling at the camera, at me. Her breasts and body are still intact. Our lives were still intact.

Yesterday as friends visited, Barbara sat in the window seat without her hat. Perhaps she is beginning to believe the many women who have told her that the shape of her head is lovely.

*Sandy*
*August 25*

Radiation began today.

*Barbara*
*September 3*

The side effects of radiation are extremely unpleasant, enervating, creeping in slowly and catching me unaware. I'm exhausted, but it's different from the exhaustion of chemotherapy. A different depletion, different sense of lassitude.

There is a terrible lump in my throat all the time. And it seems the only way to get rid of it is by swallowing. Yet swallowing is painful and hurts my throat even more. A cycle of pain and swallowing, swallowing and pain. My mouth is always full of saliva: the more I get nervous, the more I produce; the more I swallow, the more it hurts, the more I get nervous. All my throat muscles are in spasm, complicating whatever is going on in my esophagus.

My concentration is focused and deliberate. I need to get through radiation, with its fatigue and the terrible pain in my throat.

*Barbara*
*September 8*

The malpractice suit is looming in just a few weeks and my lawyer expects the arbitration to be tough. She needs to take many depositions and I have to hear details of the medical mistakes that were made that led to my shortened life. I will have to get a new CAT brain scan and have the old one reread.

I know there is a point, an important point to this fight. It's about women's bodies. It's a struggle to overcome negligence and incompetence. I try to remember.

*Barbara*
*September 9*

To have a cylindrical machine pointed at me, scanning me, is a terrifying experience, filling me with foreboding. The strain is unbearable. These machines with penetrating calibrating vision are the ultimate arbiters of truth. To engage with them is as emotion-laden as consulting the oracle.

Waiting is agony. Waiting for the machine to mechanically scan the body. Turn to the left. Move to the right. Don't move. Hold your breath. Relax. Undergoing the procedure feels like a form of torture I don't understand.

Lying there stiffly, I weep.

When the procedure is completed, there is still the waiting time for interpretation. Are my lungs clear? Is there contamination in my bones? What about that pain in my elbow? My dizziness seems to be returning. It diminishes when I'm on chemotherapy but now I'm frightened that the cancer has metastasized to my brain. Is there evidence of more cancer?

I wait with Sandy, full of anxiety, heart beating hard and fast, until relief comes. "No, there's no cancer anywhere else that is currently detectable using this technology," the doctor says in the guarded language of diagnosis.

It's not enough, but it's all there is.


*Barbara*
*September 11*

The effects of radiation are terrible now and there is nonstop itching on the entire surface of my skin. I don't know who scratches more, my dog Sembei with her fleas or me with my burnt skin.


*Sandy*
*September 12*

I feel a pervasive sense of weariness. A heaviness presses against me, requiring more and more doggedness to lift, even for a few hours.

Each night I awake tantalized by rich, voluptuous images, phrases that shatter and disappear if I try to rise and write them down. This morning I went to my desk and saw scrawled in thick red pen, nearly the same color as the markings on Barbara's chest, the words, "I long—I long." I don't remember waking up, writing it down or, more importantly, what it was I longed for in the night. My appetites feel consuming, engulfing. Just below them lie the terror, the fear of abandonment, the roaring of grief and of muffled rage. How much acceptance of despair is a necessary part of the acceptance of living?


*Barbara*
*September 13*

Sandy is away again and I miss her very much. And I love her very much. I'm proud of the work we are doing together. Suffering is ordinary.

My parents have come back to San Francisco to be with me during the last ten days of radiation. They walk so cutely together, arms linked. My father steadies my mother—her arthritis makes walking difficult. She helps him see, his increasing blindness making navigating curbs and traffic harrowing. Their presence is wonderful. They make me feel good, peaceful, optimistic. My mother reassured me that the cancer won't come back and I believe her. A kind of belief, despite my knowing the statistics, the probabilities, the chances.

And now there are a dozen containers of homemade soup in the freezer.

*Sandy*
*September 18*

VANCOUVER. I have been working here for four days while Barbara's parents are at home with her. It seems hard for her to reach out to me, perhaps because her parents are there, perhaps because time has taken on such urgency. She talks now about having the house to herself more often, about writing, about wanting to travel with friends.

I admire and respect her tenaciousness and dignity in the face of this disease. Her loyalty to friends. Her protectiveness and love for her parents and sister. But my need to be central in her life feels overwhelming and I flounder in this new role. I feel isolated, lonely.

*Barbara*
*September 18*

When we are all together, I am relaxed, part of a system. But when first Sandy and then my parents left, I had tremendous separation anxiety. I felt like a seal or a baboon that's been separated from its mother. If I could, I would make those heartbreaking animal sounds that reach the deepest places of the soul to express my longing.

*Barbara*
*September 20*

Sandy is home now and we have begun to talk about preparing my legal and medical power of attorney. Clear talk, realistic, no bullshit. Anyhow, I've got a life to live, whatever its length.

Fall is in the air; the tomatoes are mature. Time for planting a winter garden. A quiet takes over. I must endure this radiation and following that, the arbitration, and following that, a year of chemotherapy. I will try to endure: with fortitude, with perseverance, with guts. With good cheer.

*Sandy*
*September 28*

We celebrated the end of radiation last week. The skin across her chest appears sunburned, red, and bubbly, and Barbara creams it every day with aloe. The image of her lying beneath the massive radiation machine, staring up at the ceiling while being zapped with poison, is permanently traced in my brain. Her indefatigable good spirits are as well.

The lawsuit is scheduled to begin soon and I am determined that "they" be held responsible for their shoddy medicine, their indifference. One doctor said in his deposition that he had met Barbara but he never did. Another lied about the wording of his report of the mammogram results. I will never forget the sound of his disembodied voice on our phone machine saying, "The mammo is clear but if you are still worried, go see a surgeon." He now insists he said, "Be sure to see a surgeon"—which, of course, Barbara would have done. Their goddamn cavalier attitudes. The hasty examinations, inadequate information, and incorrect diagnosis. The way in which Barbara fell through the cracks of the system is intolerable to me.

But I know it's not just Barbara. Women should not be blamed, underserved, invisible, alone. Barbara isn't now, and no woman should ever be. Women have built movements before. We can do it again.

*Sandy*
*September 30*

Now I want to look ahead. To the end of chemo, radiation, lawsuits. To remission of whatever length. To a sort of dailiness that eludes us now. Everything is heightened, carries immediacy, feels portentous. Barbara and I went to Temple Sha'ar Zahav for *Yom Kippur*, the Day of Atonement, the most sacred of the Holy Days, and sobbed throughout the service. Both of us so raw, so unprotected. All our feelings on the surface now.

Barbara's bald head drew curious stares, many in our gay and lesbian congregation wondering if she had AIDS or cancer and was taking chemotherapy. Breast cancer strikes one in nine women now. The men and the women in this congregation, each with our own epidemic.

Now a business trip to Huntington and Little Rock, timed to coincide with Barbara's faculty meeting in Vermont. Our home empties as we ascend in planes taking us to different parts of the country. Barbara seems glad for the distraction of the meetings, the pleasure of a few old friends in Boston, the fall colors. She seems less anxious about the upcoming litigation and more thoughtful about the many and complex meanings of her upcoming tenure review.

*Barbara*
*October 1*

A fine spray coats the air, the trees are in half-silhouette against the strange lightness of this fog, punctuated by a yellow accent of an autumn leaf that pierces through the mist, as I write in my journal before a faculty meeting.

There are seven dead flies on the floor, this room is airless and stale, my nose is stuffy and I have a million feelings simmering beneath the surface. I'm lonely and sad on this balmy night. I wish Sandy were here. I miss her soothing body next to mine, and the comfort of Sembei in the next room. I miss my garden and my home. I miss my mother and father and feel panicky that I have not been able to reach them on the phone. I'm very weepy and melancholy about my limitations.

All my life I wanted to be a tenured university professor. I had the outsider's romantic vision of tweed jackets, heather sweaters, blazing sunsets. A fireplace with a good book and music afterwards. Tenure. The stamp of legitimacy. The guarantee of lifetime employment and a pension for retirement.

I went up for tenure once and was so shattered by the process and its outcome that I did a 180 degree turn and took an academic job in a nontraditional program that eschewed the entire system. But now they too have instituted tenure, after all that ideological idealism.

Tenure is a ranked system of statuses, a hierarchy of offices through which one moves. It begins in graduate school, which is oversupplied with excellent people, many of whom, for one reason or another, cannot or will not make it in academia. Candidates are continuously weeded out. Some get prized fellowships. Others get prime jobs in universities. Most don't.

The neophyte teaches, writes, publishes, gets grants, makes connections, becomes visible, and learns the politics of being properly mentored in a department. For females, having an older male advocate is still traditional, like the father giving away the bride. The same is true for men, who have always performed this function for each other.

Tenure is a peculiar form of social organization that mixes aspects of mobility with those of kinship. The young ones of the tribe fiercely compete for the prize, for who will be one of the next generation's carriers of knowledge. They are evaluated on the basis of three factors—magnitude, velocity, and quality. The amount one publishes is not enough. It must be evaluated in terms of the trajectory of time. And quality, too, that elusive ingredient.

The initiation process consists of a series of tests the candidate has to pass. As in most initiations, she must show courage and strength, especially in such ceremonial rituals as prelims, orals, and job searches. In a system that emphasizes criticism, attack, and counterattack, the neophyte must learn to defend herself against competition-induced behaviors like one-upmanship. Because it is based on a zero-sum game, where one's status is diminished by someone else's good performance, the candidate must show decorum and cool where others might get rattled, upset, argumentative, or lose control. The ethos of "good work" runs concurrently with the norms of "good performance." Not only should one's work be empirically sound, theoretically sophisticated, and tightly reasoned, it helps enormously if the presentation is witty, clever, entertaining, written with such rhetorical devices as an in joke or an elegant turn of phrase. Camouflaged and cloistered in the niceties of genteel discourse, the academic attack and counterattack argument can be just as vicious as tribal warfare. In an ongoing series of battles, the initiate shows elders and peers that she is made of the right stuff—that she can survive in their world.

Then after a seven-year trial period, the elders make their judgment. Those who succeed are given a permanent place and the rules that previously defined their efforts are no longer applicable. Instead, one's rights and obligations change. There are new roles: that of the media spokesperson, the grant entrepreneur, the administrative head. There are new rules, rules of kinship and belonging, a sense of community, and responsibility to fairly share the tasks that must be performed by these elders.

This year, the same year as my diagnosis, the same year I learned I have five years left to live, I will be given tenure. I will die knowing I have arrived, obtained peer and elder approval—knowing I am made of the right stuff. A bittersweet lifetime guarantee.

*Barbara*
*October 8*

I feel crazed! At 8 a.m. yesterday, an ordinary morning, I was out at a construction site gathering irregularly shaped blocks of scrap wood for the fireplace in my office.

Just three and a half hours later everything was changed. I was sitting in my lawyer's office listening to the phone call which radically changed my post-diagnosis life. Kaiser settled my case before trial for $296,000 plus $25,000 a year, increasing 3 percent annually for the length of my life. Which makes me very rich.

*Barbara*
*October 25*

This is the most discombobulating thing that has ever happened to me. When I got the diagnosis, my first impulse was to reach out to people. To be close. To connect with people I loved. Now there are secrets. I am advised not to tell anyone. Not to talk about the dollar amount. I feel pressures to support this organization or that family member. There are gifts I want to give.

The most unsettling thing about all of this is that I'm a person who rarely has had fantasies. Now I feel so ungrounded and have spending fantasies every other minute. Travel, research assistants, books, art work, gifts to my family, investments. Even more so because the money from Kaiser is just for me. Between Kaiser and Vermont College's insurance, most of my medical bills will be paid for separately.

I've been on tranquilizers to try to calm down. Ordinary life—going to the office, reading—helps to quiet this ongoing panicky feeling.

*Sandy*
*October 26*

It's been just a few weeks since Barbara's settlement and my feelings fill me with anxiety and confusion. My hand feels heavy as I write. A price tag on Barbara's life.

I walk on the university campus in South Dakota, and the barren trees, the feel of the air on my skin, evoke the bleak landscape of New England after the leaves have fallen, the ground hard and closed. Everything poised for the first snow. And I feel like the girl I once was, walking home from elementary school, little and lonesome, waiting for winter.

When I was that child, all "naughtiness" was punished in the same way. My allowance was cut off. All good grades or good behavior was rewarded with a present. Money was the currency of emotions.

I have never accumulated money and always gave it away when I had even a bit more than I needed. Now Barbara wants to spend this new money on herself. On her family. On me. But for me to have money means I am no longer myself. I will become my mother. A woman with money.

My father, during his final years, felt like a failure about not having accumulated "enough" money and was (perhaps like his own father) unable to see and enjoy what he had. Money was always the arbiter of success for him.

Somehow all this makes me feel I was robbed. Betrayed by Barbara's cancer. Unable to identify the thief—wondering if something was my fault. If I was bad or undeserving. Not destined for riches I really wanted. Having money instead.

And then there's my confusion about all this money. Is it ours? Hers? Do I want to be consulted about its distribution? What would it feel like to be supported? Part of me yearns to be taken care of in that way, but even my mother cautions me not to lose my life in Barbara's, much as she was lost in my father's. I haven't been a wife in over twenty-five years but can imagine myself having time to fix fresh flowers for the table, prepare nourishing meals, take long walks, travel together. I want to come to rest alongside Barbara now—to make a nest for us, sit quietly in our yard, cherishing her and the time we have left. Such dependency frightens me even as I long for it.

*Sandy*
*October 30*

Last night I wrote, "I am excused. I excuse myself. Cancer is what I do now." Cancer is my work. Barbara's mood swings, doctor's appointments, medicines. My feelings. Our writing together. All of it has become my central activity. Cancer swallows up the air of my life and insinuates its presence everywhere. Nothing remains untouched. Inviolate.

So I am excused. I don't want to be separate now. Time is too valuable. I will be separate soon enough. I am excused. I excuse myself from autonomy. I need now to yield, to allow the dependence on this woman who has become my life.

*Barbara*
*October 30*

With all this focus on the medical malpractice suit and financial settlement, I have lost a quiet center. There are too many people in my life now. Doctors, lawyers, financial advisers. It's time to get back to quiet. To read, write book reviews, work with students, go to the opera. Time to think. It is so noisy and quivery inside me.

The ironies of blood money are deeper than I ever imagined. No one would trade money for what I have to go through. Money is nothing. I never wanted it. If I had wanted money, I would have worked for it in some business or corporation. I would have learned money management and public relations skills, like how to build motivation or morale. At least, I would have learned bookkeeping.

No. I wanted time. Time to read and to think, to walk my dog. (I thought at one time, to have a child.) Time to contemplate the intense orange of a persimmon. Time to take pictures. To argue with other thinkers. To cut wood for the fireplace.

I don't have so much time anymore. The horizon line of my life comes in closer and closer. A day is so precious. I want to cram everything into it.

That's the way the system works. Redress for grievances. But in my soul, my heart, it rings horribly of a Faustian pact with the devil. This money in exchange for years of my life. $1,000 for every vomit. $1,000 for every cut, every needle in my arm. Every gag. Every wave of nausea. Every hurt, pain, and ache in my body. Every nosebleed. Every anguished moment. No sane person would make such a contract.

*Sandy*
*November 4*

Barbara's mother fell and is in the hospital with a broken hip. Her father, blind and diabetic, is unable to give himself his necessary daily insulin shots because he cannot see which vial is empty and which is full. Their dependency on each other. My dependency on Barbara.

*Barbara*
*November 5*

NEW YORK. Last week, my mother fell, broke her hip, was hospitalized and is now having physical therapy. No one called me for days. My father didn't tell me when we spoke on the phone; my sister left messages to call but never said why. I'm angry at everyone but, most of all, I feel like a nine-year-old child again. This is the worst, hardest to deal with, not being included. Being lied to.

And I see, sadly, that I recapitulated the lying they did to me—the secret of my mother's depression and electroshock therapy when I was nine—when I kept the seriousness of my cancer from them. All in the stupid name of protection from hurt, sparing the other, not understanding that the despair of exclusion and isolation is far more of a burden than the truth.

I have a much deeper understanding of family secrets and I am very sad. I also feel incredibly helpless, imagining my mother's pain. I have never felt so close and bonded to her as in these last months, since I told her I have cancer. With the telling came the closeness. A closeness that has been sitting inside of me, burning for forty years. I feel so tied to her, so corded, so umbilically connected.

*Barbara*
*November 9*

I feel numb. My father is in the hospital now with a mild heart attack; my mother hobbling around on a walker. And I am here in Brooklyn, between the second and third round of chemotherapy cycles, to help them. Still and always the oldest daughter.

I make daily trips to Coney Island Hospital, talk to the doctors, take my mother to the surgeon, and all the while, try to remain cheerful and cope with everything. That's all I do, it seems. Cope.

I have displaced affect this week—the kind where I cry at television sentimentality or stare in awe at a photograph on a book about Yosemite, but see my own mother's face as ordinary.

Yesterday I watched my father sleeping and imagined he was dead and I was at his funeral. His face, flaccid, looked so different. It made me aware of his aliveness, his animation, his life force present in his constantly changing and expressive face. Later I looked at my mother sleeping. She seems peaceful, the medical report good. Her prognosis is excellent and she's ready for a quad cane. Today was long and difficult, her first day out in weeks, but she did wonderfully. She even dressed up for the occasion!

My heart breaks at the thought of leaving them to return home. Separation anxiety. Guilt. It weighs me down, so much that I can barely imagine being light enough to fly. Just to be able to cope. To handle everything.

# A Woman Dead
# in Her Forties

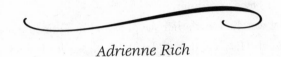

*Adrienne Rich*

1.

Your breasts/ sliced-off  The scars
dimmed   as they would have to be
years later

All the women I grew up with are sitting
half-naked on rocks   in sun
we look at each other and
are not ashamed

and you too have taken off your blouse
but this was not what you wanted:

to show your scarred, deleted torso

I barely glance at you

as if my look could scald you
though I'm the one who loved you

I want to touch my fingers
to where your breasts had been
but we never did such things

You hadn't thought everyone
would look so perfect
unmutilated

you pull on
your blouse again:   stern statement:

*There are things I will not share
with everyone*

2.
You send me back to share
my own scars   first of all
with myself

What did I hide from her
what have I denied her
what losses suffered

how in this ignorant body
did she hide

waiting for her release
till uncontrollable light began to pour

from every wound and suture
and all the sacred openings

3.
Wartime.   We sit on warm
weathered, softening grey boards

the ladder glimmers where you told me
the leeches swim

I smell the flame
of kerosene   the pine

boards where we sleep side by side
in narrow cots

the night-meadow exhaling
its darkness   calling

child into woman
child into woman
woman

4.
Most of our love from the age of nine
took the form of jokes and mute

loyalty:   you fought a girl
who said she'd knock me down

we did each other's homework
wrote letters   kept in touch, untouching

lied about our lives:   I wearing
the face of the proper marriage

you the face of the independent woman

We cleaved to each other across that space

fingering webs
of love and estrangement   till the day

the gynecologist touched your breast
and found a palpable hardness

5.
You played heroic, necessary
games with death

since in your neo-protestant tribe the void
was supposed not to exist

except as a fashionable concept
you had no traffic with

I wish you were here tonight   I want
to yell at you

*Don't accept*
*Don't give in*

But would I be meaning your brave
irreproachable life, you dean of women, or

your unfair, unfashionable, unforgivable
woman's death?

6.
You are every woman I ever loved
and disavowed

a bloody incandescent chord strung out
across years, tracts of space

How can I reconcile this passion
with our modesty

your calvinist heritage
my girlhood frozen into forms

how can I go on this mission
without you

you, who might have told me
*everything you feel is true?*

7.
Time after time in dreams you rise
reproachful

once from a wheelchair pushed by your father
across a lethal expressway

Of all my dead it's you
who come to me unfinished

You left me amber beads
strung with turquoise from an Egyptian grave

I hear them wondering
How am I true to you?

I'm half-afraid to write poetry
for you   who never read it much

and I'm left laboring
with the secrets and the silence

In plain language:   I never told you how I loved you
we never talked at your deathbed of your death

8.
One autumn evening in a train
catching the diamond-flash of sunset

in puddles along the Hudson
I thought:   *I understand*

*life and death now, the choices*
I didn't know your choice

or how by then you had no choice
how the body tells the truth in its rush of cells

Most of our love took the form
of mute loyalty

*we never spoke at your deathbed of your death*

but from here on
I want more crazy mourning, more howl, more keening

We stayed mute and disloyal
because we were afraid

I would have touched my fingers
to where your breasts had been
but we never did such things

# KNOW YOUR BODY, SAVE YOUR LIFE
## An Interview with Kelly Marbury

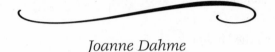

*Joanne Dahme*

KELLY MARBURY FEELS THREATENED. She is in the middle of radiation treatment for breast cancer and has just completed chemotherapy. Her prognosis is good and her body seemed to recover quickly from the chemo, although she still experiences lingering side effects and doesn't quite feel like her precancer self. The threat that cancer posed to Kelly felt like the evil of a man with a knife in a dark alley. Something scary and unexpected intruded on her life, and she still feels violated by it. She knew the documented stages of coping with trauma: first, denial when you are diagnosed and put through the rigors of treatment. But later, after the chemo is almost completed, it hits you: Your life has been threatened in a way that it was never threatened before. When treatment ends, it hits again, like a recurring flashback. Kelly now says she feels as if adrenaline and medication are the forces that are keeping her going.

Kelly is a young black woman—thirty-six years old—quite young to be diagnosed with cancer. Statistically, cancer was not supposed to be on her mind—she was too young to have yearly mammograms—so what led to her diagnosis? "During sleep, exercise and trips to the chiropractor, I found that it was difficult to be flat on my stomach because my breasts hurt too much from the pressure. I do routine breast self-examinations. I started feeling lumps in both breasts." Her gynecologist suggested a mammogram because Kelly's breasts are quite large and she had felt the lumps, too. The results of the first mammogram were rather unremarkable, except for the cluster of calcifications in Kelly's right breast. The report from the radiologist noted that these clusters were "probably benign."

"My gynecologist recommended one thousand milligrams of vitamin E once a day and told me to avoid caffeine. This helped with both the lumps and the tenderness. She also recommended another mammogram in six months and suggested that I see a surgeon sometime in the future." Kelly had the second mammogram. The technician told her to wait because the radiologist wanted to look at something on the x-ray from the right breast (the one with the calcifications). A few minutes later, Kelly met the radiologist. He wanted to take a closer look by way of a sonogram. Afterward, the radiologist looked at Kelly and then said, "You need to see a surgeon immediately."

Kelly found a breast surgeon who aspirated what appeared to be a cyst. The cyst then seemed to disappear. Kelly's surgeon sent her for another mammogram and some close-ups of the calcifications and the area he aspirated. An hour after the surgeon aspirated the cyst, however, it became quite clear that whatever the thing was, it was back to stay. "My surgeon and I decided that he would take out the thing and have a pathologist decide if it was benign or malignant. My surgeon called the next day to say the thing was indeed cancer."

Kelly's prognosis is good, although she has a rare form of breast cancer called medullary cancer, which comprises only ten percent of all breast cancer cases. Of all forms of breast cancer, this is the most favorable as far as treatment and prognosis are concerned. Because medullary breast cancer is so rare, the research and treatment protocol is based on the more common forms of breast cancer. The tumor that was removed was three centimeters, stage-two diagnosis because of the size, which meant that Kelly needed four cycles of chemotherapy. Before she knew she would have to undergo chemotherapy, Kelly already decided on a lumpectomy and thirty-three days of radiation treatment.

The available statistics on black women with cancer are not heartening, there is often a later diagnosis, a lack of comprehensive treatment and higher death rates. Kelly hopes that things are changing in this regard. "The tumor that was removed grew very quickly. If I didn't do routine breast self-examinations, I would have never known there were changes in my breast, and the cancer would have spread to other organs. It probably would have killed me if I didn't know my body and I wasn't proactive in seeking medical attention at the first sign of something feeling wrong."

The statistics did not frighten Kelly as far as her diagnosis, treatment and prognosis were concerned. Over the course of treatment, she has read about or met many black women who are breast cancer survivors, which led Kelly to believe that as a group black women are now getting screened more frequently for cancer. Kelly still feels strongly, however, that women, especially black women, need to stay in touch with their bodies. "I am young. I've never lived near a toxic waste dump. I do not smoke. I do not drink excessive amounts of alcohol. I exercise regularly and have a firm grip on getting the stresses of life under control. I have been a strict vegetarian for almost ten years and try to eat only organic foods. I am the first woman in my family with breast cancer."

Kelly counts herself as one of the blessed in a world new to her marked by adversity and pain. As soon as her mother, Sharlene, learned about Kelly's diagnosis, she left her home in San Diego to join Kelly in Takoma Park, Maryland, to help her through chemotherapy and to accompany Kelly to all of her doctor's appointments. Sharlene was no stranger to cancer. Kelly's dad, Richard, had died ten years earlier from a rare stomach cancer. Already terminal when diagnosed, he died nine months later. Sharlene, therefore, knew what to expect from Kelly's chemo, although she was amazed by how much the treatment has changed for the better. She was thankful that the side effects of chemo are substantially less devastating than they were years ago. Sharlene has since returned to San Diego as Kelly's treatment is drawing to a close.

Kelly has also received much support from the Washington, D.C., area lesbian community and from the Mary-Helen Mautner Project for Lesbians with Cancer. She also became involved with the Lesbian Services program at the Whitman-Walker Clinic, through which Kelly met a diverse lesbian community via participation in the peer support and rap group team. Kelly joined the Lesbian Services steering committee and became the support group coordinator because she thought this was a positive way to give her time and energies to the community. This personal investment proved more valuable than gold. Kelly's battle with breast cancer has not been a lonely one, as her friends in the lesbian community have rallied around her. Kelly is extremely grateful for the support provided by the Mautner Project, whose knowledgeable and sensitive staff assisted her in the quest to learn all she needed to know to fight her breast cancer. Although the staff was willing, she didn't need them to accompany her on doctor's visits because her mother was available. However, they provided plenty of informational and emotional support. "Besides the kind words, offers for breakfast and rubs on the head from women I barely know, I've received the help and support of Mautner in the following areas: rides to medical appointments, shopping for groceries, companion animal care, lawn care, massages, meals, running errands and providing relief for my mom." In fact, one of the project's volunteers discovered that Sharlene shared similar shopping interests, and soon, the Mautner volunteer and her partner were coming by every weekend to take Sharlene along on their excursions.

Kelly had been aware of the Mautner Project before her own diagnosis. Her friend, Susan Hester happens to be the client services director of Mautner. Kelly had been approached by Susan and Kathleen DeBold, the executive director of Mautner, to speak at a fundraiser about the project and her own experiences with breast cancer. A friendship was fast developing between Kelly and Kathleen. Kelly is not currently an "official" volunteer for the Mautner Project in the sense that she hasn't gone through the formal training that the project provides for volunteers who wish to give one-on-one support for clients. However, she has been volunteering her professional marketing skills to write fundraising letters and other informational materials since December 1999. (Kelly is a marketer for a company that develops software for not-for-profit organizations.) She began volunteering right around the time she began her last round of chemotherapy. By offering her marketing services, Kelly insists that this is her "tiny way of repaying the project for all of the support they have given her" since her August 1999 diagnosis. Her goal is to "do something and speak out on behalf of the project, to get more volunteers on behalf of the project" an important component in Kelly's own battle against breast cancer.

Now undergoing radiation treatments, Kelly says the radiation is not painful, although it does cause a sunburn and skin dryness. She explains that the radiation treatment, when compared with the chemo, is thankfully "boring, although it tends to sap all of your energies." Boring can be a good thing, Kelly asserts, as she enumerates the positive things in her life. Topping the list is her mother, who has always been incredibly supportive and who has made it clear to Kelly that she is the most important thing in her mother's life. Kelly also cites her terrific medical team. Her surgeon was more than Kelly could have hoped for, recommended her to a "fabulous" oncologist, never mentioning the fact that this oncologist was a black woman and one of the top in her profession in the Washington, D.C.–Baltimore area. This was amazing to Kelly, as a woman of color herself. Kelly's employer and her "incredibly x" co-workers have also been extremely supportive. The final quarter of the year is usually the slow time for the businesses, so it wasn't as difficult for Kelly to take time off for chemo treatment and recovery. She has also been able to work at home, and one of her co-workers has been picking up her travel duties.

Sometimes Kelly feels as if she is still in the trenches, however. She is frustrated that she hasn't started exercising again. Also, her appetite is not quite normal, although she is eating well-balanced meals. When she sees something red, though, it reminds her of the chemo medication and it makes her stomach queasy. Any shade close to that dark red color, or the color of blood, still freaks her out. Even the clear saline solution of an IV makes Kelly lose her appetite. She trusts that this is temporary, and she is already thinking about options for her future. Has cancer caused Kelly to look at life in a different way? Is she more interested in relationships than her job, more spiritual, less apt to let life's smaller challenges upset her? "I'm kind of still in the denial phase since I'm still being treated for the thing formerly known as my tumor. I'm currently at the six months after diagnosis point and can only now pick up anything related to breast cancer. Amazingly enough, however, I'm not self-conscious about my body or the effect that cancer might have on future relationships. I've been walking around with my bald head for a month—and getting more attention than when I had curly-wavy locks of hair that bounced halfway down my back."

Kelly is originally from a small town outside of Pittsburgh, Pennsylvania, and has lived in the Washington, D.C., area for twenty years. But now she is pondering a move. Her mom and her best friend both live in San Diego, so she is thinking seriously about moving out there in a few years to perhaps open up a new life. Kelly is an only child and her mother would be thrilled to have her nearby. As Kelly does not have a special partner in her life at this time, she feels that perhaps all signs are pointing her west. The breast cancer may have been disorienting, but Kelly believes that she now controls the compass to her life.

# Murder at the
# Nightwood Bar

*Katherine V. Forrest*

KATE LEFT THE STATION SHORTLY after ten o'clock. As she threaded her way through the downtown freeway interchange and over quiet city streets to the Silverlake District, persistent waves of fatigue encroached on her anticipation of time alone with Andrea. The day had been long, beginning with the autopsy of Dory Quillin and ending with the paperwork she had had to complete at the station. But it was the confrontation in the parking lot of the Nightwood Bar, the full expenditure of adrenaline, which had so depleted her.

The house was a small white frame, its old-fashioned veranda dark and shadowy with the shapes of leafy plants. Kate frowned at the flimsy aluminum-frame door, the light, easily removable screens and windows. A two-year-old could break into this place. Disturbed, she rang the bell.

From the backyard a dog snarled, then barked. Kate was suddenly bathed in light which illuminated the forest of plants on the veranda. To her relief, the light also revealed a substantial inside door and a barred living room window. The house was not nearly as vulnerable as it appeared.

Andrea, in jeans and a large blue plaid shirt, stood framed in the inner doorway, her house warm brightness behind her; then she came out onto the veranda to unlock the door. The rich aroma of coffee reached Kate. She felt suddenly weak with the womanly presence of Andrea and the warmth of her house; she ached with tiredness and loneliness.

"You look exhausted," Andrea said, taking her arm, leading her into the living room. "How about something stronger than coffee?"

"Coffee is fine." Kate sank into a thickly cushioned sofa, and looked curiously around her. As if the veranda had overflowed into this room, plants occupied the floor and the slate hearth of a fireplace, as well as the surfaces of the glass-topped coffee table, two cherrywood occasional tables, several shelves of a tall bookcase. On the wall across from her hung a large print, geometric bands of color, costly-looking in its simplicity. The room had been put together with care, and Kate felt comfortable in it.

"Is it that you don't drink at all?" Andrea inquired. "Surely you can't still be on duty. Do they work police officers eighteen hours a day?"

"On a homicide investigation we don't have set hours. We have to move fast, develop information fast. We go till we can't go any longer. So I'm still on duty. Technically, I have no business being here unless I *am* on duty."

"Okay, you're on duty. Now what would you like to drink on duty? I have some excellent brandy, also scotch, vodka, wine—you look like a scotch drinker to me."

Kate smiled. "You're very observant. And kind. Right now some coffee with a little brandy sounds perfect."

Andrea disappeared into the kitchen. Kate pulled an ottoman over from the end of the sofa, feeling at ease about doing so, and kicked off her shoes and put her feet up.

Andrea came back carrying two mugs of steaming coffee and placed them on the coffee table. From a cabinet in the bottom of the bookcase she took a bottle of Henessey and two bubble glasses, and poured generously.

"All the plants you have in here, they're wonderful," Kate commented, accepting the snifter of brandy, warming it in both hands.

"Plants are easily the healthiest life forms on this earth," Andrea said forcefully. "They don't prey on one another, and you can keep them alive and growing forever."

"I never thought about them that way," Kate murmured, surprised by the intensity in Andrea's voice. The first sip of brandy was ambrosial, the liquor easing its silky way through her tiredness.

"Anything new on the three neanderthals?" Gracefully, Andrea seated herself next to Kate, tucking her feet under her, her glass of brandy cupped in a palm.

"They all have rap sheets. Burglary, sale of stolen property. No drugs on them, there may be some in the car. But most dopers don't stockpile unless they're dealing, they can't afford to. They ingest whatever they buy."

"Real assets to society," Andrea said dourly.

Kate swallowed coffee that was strong and bracing. "I can tell you what their story will be tomorrow when we question them. That Audie offered to go with them and you women at the bar interfered and I, prejudiced woman cop that I am, wronged them. We'll question them within an inch of their lives about Dory, of course."

"Kate—young men like those three, surely they don't all end up in prison, there are too many. What happens when they grow up?"

"*If* they grow up," Kate amended. "Maybe one of the three—"

The phone rang. On the second ring it clicked into an answering machine.

"*Andy honey I know you're there, please pick up the phone . . .*" The woman's voice came softly from the speaker, tremulous with need. "*Andy . . . pick up the phone, baby . . . please . . .*"

Andrea walked over to the answering machine, turned the volume off. "You were saying," she said to Kate.

Kate swallowed more coffee. "Maybe one of them will find a good person to marry," she continued, watching Andrea as she settled herself once more on the sofa. "But a felony record is death in the job market, and he'll never have a job of any consequence. Maybe he'll scratch along in the underground economy, maybe he won't."

Andrea's eyes were fixed on the answering machine; its message-waiting light had not yet begun to blink, indicating that the caller was still speaking.

"More likely," Kate continued, "they'll all end up dealing drugs. Maybe get caught, do serious jail time. They'll probably die young—an overdose or a drug-related failure of some vital organ. Or their brains will get so fried they'll become wandering zombies living out of garbage cans."

The message-waiting light finally began to blink, Andrea's eyes still fastened on it. Kate doubted that she had heard a single word she had said. "Andrea," she asked, "is someone bothering you?"

Andrea's eyes, cool and expressionless, met hers. "My ex-lover. She calls all the time. Thanks to my answering machine, I never have to talk to her."

Her senses invaded by the subtle scent of perfume, the beauty of Andrea's face and bearing, Kate looked at her in a warmth of desire. Whatever could this ex-lover have done to earn such enmity from Andrea?

Kate cleared her throat. "I was wondering, I thought perhaps . . . " She had spoken impulsively, and now she sorted through frantic thoughts: What could she invite Andrea to do? She was unable to cook a decent dinner, a movie seemed too juvenile. "Depending on what happens with this case, I'm free this weekend. I thought perhaps . . . Maybe you'd like to have dinner at the beach—" She broke off, confused by the hardening grimness in Andrea's face.

"I was quite certain you were attracted to me." The voice was flat, almost accusatory.

Confounded by Andrea's tone, Kate put down her coffee mug and tried to gather her wits. "I—I'm sure I have that in common with a lot of women."

"You're wasting your time, Kate." The words were bitten off. "I'm not at all what I seem."

"In what way?" She was completely bewildered.

But Andrea did not reply. Closing her eyes, she lifted her brandy snifter and took a deep swallow.

"I go by instinct," Kate said, desperate to bring this conversation into the realm of comprehension. "I learned to do that in police work and I've relied on it—I've had to. You're one of the most interesting and attractive women I've met in a long time. In every way."

"Every way?" Andrea was unbuttoning the cuffs of her shirt.

"Every way," Kate confirmed, still groping to locate solid ground somewhere.

Andrea seized the tails of her shirt in both hands and tugged it up and over her head.

Kate stared at two red scars making their jagged and lengthy way across a puffy expanse of dusky flesh, the scars neatly and evenly cross-hatched by pink stitch marks.

"See how deceiving appearances can be?" Andrea's voice was soft; she did not look at Kate. She continued almost inaudibly, "My breasts used to be larger than yours."

Kate reached to her, needing to protect the rawness of those scars, needing to protect Andrea's nakedness from the coolness of this green room. She grasped Andrea's bare shoulders to warm her, rubbing, chafing the cool flesh under her hands, and looked into eyes that stared in amazement into hers.

"Listen to me," Kate said quietly. "The woman I loved burned to death a year and ten months ago. I would have taken her without arms or legs or breasts. I would have taken her with burns or scars or anything—if only Anne could have lived."

Andrea buried her face in Kate's shoulder.

Kate took her into her arms, moved her hands over the soft flesh of Andrea's back. "It's all right. Andrea, you're beautiful still. It's all right."

"I'm not," Andrea whispered. "What Bev said was true."

Bev—the woman on the phone? Andrea's former lover? "What did she say?" Kate drew her close.

"Nothing. Nothing at all."

"I don't understand. When was this?"

Andrea's voice was muffled against the fabric of Kate's jacket. "Four months after . . . the surgery. I hadn't looked at myself, not even when the bandages came off. I . . . couldn't."

Andrea lifted her head to gaze again at Kate, her brown eyes glistening with tears. "I wouldn't let Bev look, either. We didn't make love, I was in pain some of the time, there was a lot of numbness . . . But mostly I couldn't stand to be touched. I felt so . . . *mutilated*. But I needed her to look at me, understand?"

"Yes," Kate said.

"I had to have her do it for both of us and tell both of us it was okay, that it was okay for me to look at myself . . . understand?"

"Yes," Kate said.

"And finally I did ask her . . . And then she didn't say anything, she just stared at me and then I looked down and I saw how hideous I was—"

"Andrea, you're still beautiful. You're a beautiful woman."

Andrea shook her head. "No. My breasts were *perfect* . . . " She picked up her shirt, dabbed at her eyes.

"When did you have the surgery?"

"Six months ago."

"Is everything okay? Are you fully recovered?"

"If you mean did they get it all, yes. The lymph nodes were clear. They tell me I'll be fine."

"How long were you and Bev together?"

"Four years."

"You could have given her a little more time—" Kate sighed. It was ludicrous, justifying the behavior of this woman she did not know, whose turf she had just invaded.

"What you said, the way you—if only Bev . . . "

"Andrea, she had as much anxiety as you. Some people just need more time to adjust. A friend of Anne's told her parents she was a lesbian. They didn't take it well—but two months later they were remorseful about how they'd reacted. Bev sounded pretty remorseful on the phone."

"Bev *is* slow to react about a lot of things, but this was different, Kate. She *knew* about this. She knew days before the surgery, all those months afterward . . . "

She had to convince Andrea, but to convince her she had to defend Bev. And the more she defended Bev . . .

"Andrea, knowing about something like this doesn't matter. I knew my mother was dying. But her actual death was a shock I hadn't begun to imagine."

Andrea was silent for some moments. "I'm so sorry about your lover," she finally said. "Anne was very lucky to have you for the time that she did."

"Thank you," Kate said simply.

Andrea unbuttoned Kate's jacket, taking her time, and pushed it off her. She slid her arms around Kate's shoulders. "Your metal buttons are cold on my scars," she said, smiling.

Kate chuckled, and picked up the shirt, draped it around Andrea's shoulders.

"It's chilly in here."

Andrea took Kate's face in her hands, looked into her eyes.

Kate's hands moved along the soft silky flesh of Andrea's arms to her shoulders, down her back. She held Andrea's eyes, knowing that with each passing moment Andrea saw more and more clearly her desire.

"You're very beautiful." Kate breathed the words; Andrea's face was nearing hers.

"Stay with me tonight," Andrea murmured against Kate's lips.


Invigorated by cool sharp shower spray, Kate wrapped herself in a towel and came into the small, dimly lit bedroom. Andrea was propped up on pillows, her hair dark and glossy against the whiteness, a sheet drawn up to her shoulders. She patted the edge of the bed next to her. Smiling, Kate obediently sat down beside her.

Andrea unwrapped the towel, dropped it to the floor, and unhurriedly surveyed her.

"What a fine big woman you are," she murmured, and took Kate's face in her warm hands. She ran her fingers into Kate's hair. "Your hair is wonderful, so soft and fine . . . " Her fingernails stroked Kate's scalp, creating waves of chilling sensation; Kate felt gooseflesh rise on her arms. Andrea's hands came to Kate's neck, circling it, her palms exploring its curving; then to Kate's shoulders, the nails again running lightly; and Kate could not suppress her shudders.

Smiling in evident self-satisfaction, Andrea took Kate's breasts in her hands, cupping them in her palms as if to weigh them. She slid her palms around and around the curving of them, and Kate closed her eyes to concentrate on the warm friction, her sensations deepening as Andrea's fingers began to sensuously knead, as a fingertip circled each nipple, then stroked across it.

Andrea sat up and pushed away the sheet covering herself, drew Kate to her. Again she took Kate's breasts in her hands, this time to fit them into her, sighing as she sinuously adjusted her own body. Kate slid her arms around the delicate slenderness of her, holding her closely, and lowered her slowly, careful to preserve the melding of their bodies.

As Andrea's body joined the entire length of hers, Kate sucked in her breath at the smooth warm silkiness of her. Andrea's hands caressed down her back, the fingernails again making her writhe; the warm hands moved over her hips, squeezing them with a proprietary roughness. Andrea's legs twined with hers; Kate felt the soft hair, the heat between Andrea's legs against her thigh.

"Your body is wonderful," Andrea whispered, looking at her out of dark, heavy-lidded eyes.

Leaning on her elbows, she held Andrea's face in her hands, gazing at her, and stroked smooth firm skin that was like ocean-polished stone warm in the sun. Inhaling the scent of musk, her desire keenly penetrating, she whispered, "God, I want you."

Andrea pulled Kate's mouth down to hers, her lips a possessive, increasing pressure until Kate felt the impress of teeth; then Andrea's lips became sensuous softness, yielding under hers, and as Kate's tongue entered her Kate was freshly pierced by desire that ascended to an altogether new plateau.

Andrea's hands in her hair held Kate's mouth to hers, Andrea's tongue met hers with light swift strokes, Andrea's body became subtly undulant under hers. Kate felt the moist heat between Andrea's legs move against her thigh, felt herself go out of control for the second time this night. Overpowered by her craving, she slid a hand down to Andrea's thighs.

Her palm cupped exquisite mossy warmth, her fingers sank into a satiny depth; and Andrea's thighs closed powerfully, imprisoning her. Too fast, Kate thought amid the ecstasy of her sensations, I'm doing everything too fast. . . . But Andrea's mouth became pure passion under hers, Andrea tightened her arms around the thickest part of Kate's back and rocked her upper body against Kate's breasts. Then she buried her face in Kate's shoulder and opened her legs, her hips churning as Kate's fingers began to move. Soon Andrea's hips surged in what Kate thought was her coming until they surged again and again and again in a tense quivering that only gradually stilled.

"So good," Andrea breathed, her body softening once more into Kate's. "Oh God, so good." Gently, she took Kate's hand away.

"Too fast, I was too—"

"I wanted you . . . God, just like that."

She rolled Kate over onto her back and lay on top of her, still breathing swiftly; Kate could feel her rapid heartbeats. Again Andrea fitted, adjusted Kate's breasts to her.

Kate saw the briefest wince of pain cross her face and asked in alarm, "Did I hurt you? Was I too rough?"

Andrea took a shuddering breath, and smiled. "Not that I noticed." She added, "Sometimes there's a little stinging around the scars—it's fleeting. They tell me it'll all be gone soon. Don't worry." Andrea closed her eyes, nestled into Kate. "You feel wonderful, your breasts are just incredible against me there."

She held Kate's head cradled in her arms. "You hardly need to apologize for anything," she said, and kissed her.

With Andrea's mouth on hers in lingering tenderness, Kate explored the satiny body lying on hers, sliding her hands slowly over the curves of Andrea's back and the richly firm hips, down her thighs and under them, slipping a savoring hand again into the moist warmth between her legs. Andrea was tracing an ear with her tongue; her hand came slowly down Kate, her palm caressing over her stomach, to her legs. Kate squeezed her eyes shut against too much sensation.

Throbbing from wetly caressing fingers, groaning with her need, Kate put Andrea beneath her again and moved urgently, Andrea's fingernails raking across her shoulders, down her shoulder blades. Kate groaned again as the fingernails raced down her spine, and she arched, pressing into Andrea, transfixed.

Her release sweet and full, she took her body slowly, contentedly from Andrea, lassitude already permeating her. "Don't let me sleep," she murmured, "I don't want to sleep."

"I have other plans for you, you rough, tough cop. . . . "

Sometime later she lay helpless, her nipples a fiercely sweet ache in Andrea's mouth, Andrea's merciless fingernails seeming to be everywhere at once. Then Andrea's fingertips were stroking lightly between her legs, and then Andrea was under her again, fused to the needful rhythms of her body.

Exhausted, murmuring contentment, too utterly replete to struggle, she sank into sleep, Andrea warmly in her arms, Andrea's face pillowed against her breasts.

# That Ribbon Around
# My Heart

*Olga R. Alvarado-Cofresi*

I THINK MY PARTNER BRUNIE thought it was a game, that winter day back in '96, when I said take off your bra, lay flat, put your arm over your head . . . no, not this one, that one. But with much seriousness, I placed my fingers over her breast, and explored, first one, then the other, hoping to find nothing at all, finding something after all.

It's nothing, the doctor said. Don't worry about it, she said. See ya in six months, she said. Did I ever suspect cancer? Did I ever think that eight months later she would be bald and nauseous and I'd be fearing for her life? No way. But I still worried.

Brunie's HMO was bought by another group, familiar doctors disappeared, new ones moved in. Six months later she saw a new doctor. This one explored her breasts, as I had done, and upon finding the lump, recommended a biopsy. Did I think cancer then? Nope.

We were planning a family then, and doing all the things we loved to do, hanging out in our living room reading fiction books in our underwear (some things never change), going to the movies, visiting our favorite restaurants, planning vacations. So many normal, insignificant daily things that we never took notice of. I don't remember what the sky looked like, or what birds were visiting our backyard those days. Was it windy? Did the air smell good? Could I hear children playing in the park nearby? I don't remember. So many things going unnoticed.

Biopsy Day went well. We prayed, we laughed, we kissed. In less than two hours, the lump was out, and so we laughed some more. Cancer schmancer! She didn't smoke nor drink, she worked out a million times a week, she was vegetarian for God's sakes. Brunie? Cancer? Noooo.

Doctors should get awards for Best Lack of Tact. A couple of days after Biopsy Day, while I was at work, the surgeon called her at home and blurted out THE TUMOR IS MALIGNANT, YOU HAVE CANCER. Everyone clap and whistle now. Please doc, take a bow.

It's amazing the enormity those words can carry. Cancer. Aaaah. Cancer = death. At least that is what I grew up believing. That is what it meant to us that day in June, it's what it meant to me. Lose her, now? Ever? Noooo. After so much emptiness, I had finally found happiness. A partner, friend, family member who completed my life, made me whole. And now it was being threatened? Please no, anyone but her, not her, not the love of my life, the angel of my soul, the beating of my heart.

There is no other way to describe it but terror. I've been held up at gunpoint before, and I didn't feel terror. Granted, I'm still a bit paranoid . . . okay, I'm very paranoid, but that's beside the point. No, I didn't feel terror that day when that shiny semi-automatic was pointed at my head. The guy yanked my necklace and ran, and then the fear set in, but I was alive, and knew I would be okay, and then the fear went away, just like he had. Cancer was a different story. It filled me with terror from the moment she called to tell me the news, and it never has really left. It never ran away.

I believe God equipped each of us to be warriors, and when in need, our armor kicks in, boom, just like that. Call it Xenability. No one ever taught me to be a caregiver, I didn't have a mother around to show me how, but somehow, between a strict father, a spiritual presence, and my God given nature, I jumped right into the role. I will take care of you. There was no getting out of that one, it was what I wanted to do. It was either that or feel sorry for her and for myself and I knew that would do neither of us any good. However, I believe I had more selfish motives than just to make her feel better. I'm a Pisces and this little fish wasn't going to let another sign move in on my partner! Out of the way Cancer, this is Pisces territory! You can call that zodiac envy.

One of the new friends I've made, thanks to cancer, is the internet. I know it sounds crazy and some people think it's the devil himself, but that is how I feel. When I needed it, it came through for me. Thanks buddy. After she called to tell me what the good doc had said, I logged on to the net and typed the words "breast cancer" in the little search box. Breast cancer was a completely foreign subject to me, and up to that point, the internet had served very little research purposes except to check movie reviews, get maps, and check out vacation spots. But to my surprise, tons and tons of links flashed before me (like over one hundred thousand) where I could just click and get detailed information on what breast cancer meant, what kind of treatment options she would be faced with, what different sizes of tumors meant, who to call for more information. Print. Print. Print. I'm sure my old office has forgiven me for having used so much of their company paper. Print. Print. Print.

A friend recommended *Dr. Susan Love's Breast Book* so I immediately went out and bought it. With that, the internet pages, plus the brochures I had requested from different cancer organizations, we became cancer experts. Then, it was only a matter of her deciding what treatment she would choose. We read about women who didn't like to get involved with making the decisions on what to do with their body, and pretty much let the doctors decide what was best for her. Thankfully, we chose to arm ourselves (there's that Xena complex again) with knowledge, and more knowledge so no one could put anything past us. I guess it's one of those control things we ARE proud of.

After doing everything I could to give her information (by keeping so busy I didn't feel my fear) I backed off and gave Brunie her space to decide what she should do. After all, it is her body. Plus, no one really knows how it feels to be in that situation unless they've been there themselves, and I wasn't. I was on the outside looking in, wondering, fearing, crying, holding it all in, whispering please don't die. Whatever she chose, I'd be ready to tackle it with her.

She opted for the most aggressive treatment and so our new life began.

First, another surgery to remove the rest of the tumor and the lymph nodes in her armpit. Before June, I didn't know what lymph nodes were or why they were hanging out around the armpit. And why they don't take the whole tumor out during the first operation is beyond me. The hospital staff let me hang out with her in the pre-op room and we had a good time in there too, and then we prayed and read our favorite verses from the Bible. It may sound corny to some folks, but for us, it was exactly what we needed to stay calm. And it worked, until she got wheeled away of course.

While she was being operated on, I was praying my little heart out in the waiting area. All those books and magazines I took to read went untouched. You know how in movies they show someone in the waiting room going through in their mind their whole time spent with their loved one while the other is being operated on? Well, it's true. This actually does happen.

I sat there and remembered how we had started out, how my hand felt in hers when we first danced together. I thought about how much we had been through, all the changes we had made together, how mean she used to be when she drank, and how absolutely wonderful she turned out to be when we stopped drinking. I thought about the safety and peace we had found in each other's arms, how so many times we had cried and grieved our past pains while the other simply caressed, loved, cried too. I thought about her smile, her energetic personality, her cute toes. I thought about the way our bodies fit perfectly when we embraced, like two pieces of a puzzle. These feelings and visions flashed before me in no particular order, but with great intensity.

God I loved her, I knew in my heart that this was the person I wanted to die next to. There was no question about it. What if . . . what if . . . terror.

During Brunie's recuperation time after the surgery, we were at home, and she was high on Percocet for the most part (I was so jealous). But she looked so vulnerable, so tired and weak. As I would look at her, I'd think, how dare cancer do this to her? They had attached this thin, plastic tube that came out from her side, in between all those bandages over her breast, which led to a little plastic container that drained liquid she wasn't supposed to accumulate. I gently emptied it over and over, day after day, and cursed cancer violently each time. I hated cancer then, more than I had hated anything in my life.

Chemotherapy wasn't as bad for her as it was for others, and for that we were both thankful. But it was still traumatizing. She still felt terribly nauseous and had to stay laying down for days afterwards. Her skin color was a strange, grayish color and her eyes lost the glow and energy they normally radiated. However, three weeks after her first treatment her hair was still on there and didn't seem like it was going to fall. We were excited!

We went away for the weekend, to one of our favorite beaches and did a lot of relaxing and talking, and bonding with nature. The beach had a whole different feel and look, more beautiful, more real than ever before. We noticed the seagulls as if seeing and hearing them for the very first time. The waves looked more interesting, more powerful and majestic. The hot sand felt wonderful on our bare feet. The sky looked fabulous. How had we missed all those interesting cloud formations before? She had a good time then, and I was grateful that she wasn't sick, nor too exhausted.

The first night there, I was laying in bed reading while she showered when I heard her gasp and say Oh my God! I ran to the bathroom to find her with a huge chunk of her beautiful, black curly hair in her hand. That night I borrowed scissors from a neighbor and cut off all the excess hair that had fallen and was just sitting there, hanging on to a thin thread of hair. Sort of how I felt we were doing. Barely hanging on sometimes. It was a quiet moment, not terribly frightening, but definitely strange. I snipped, she smiled, I hugged her, and we went out to eat. We were both grateful that this happened while we were away, and relaxed. I said a quiet thank you to heaven for giving her the strength to have handled it so well.

Afterwards, her head ached so bad she cried. She said it felt like her hair was being yanked out of her head. I applied jojoba oil (something my buddy internet had recommended) each day and night to her scalp to ease some of the pain, gently, very gently because just breathing on her hair hurt her so. It was so physically painful for her, and so emotionally painful for me. Those days were horrible, truly horrible.

After the pain ceased a bit, she finally had her hair buzz cut, almost all shaved off. To her surprise, she has a nice head! Everyone kept telling her everywhere how great she looked. She always looks great. I admired her so much. She went bald everywhere. No wigs on this woman! She had cancer and wanted everyone to know it could happen to them too. Both of us became cancer advocates at our jobs.

Summer had arrived and was quickly flying by us, a time when we normally swam in the pool everyday and drank virgin frozen drinks. Now, that was really out of the question. Most things made her want to throw up. The heat exhausted her and the chemo made her immune system weak so we stayed out of the sun for the most part, we couldn't have those sun rays zapping her body too much, lest we wanted to deal with another cancer.

Throughout that ordeal, she had handled everything quite well, but as is normal, was very scared, and had so many questions. I did what I could to calm them, but honestly, it was very difficult sometimes because while she was asking me, what if I die, I was thinking to myself, what if you die? And so many times I just had to hold her close so she would not see the tears in my eyes, or notice the lump in my throat. Our moods were on edge, up and down, happy, sad, angry, vulnerable, cold, and finally we got to each other. We needed help. We needed to find other people to talk to.

We had considered going to some of the support groups offered by many cancer organizations and local hospitals, but opted not to because we feared being treated as outsiders because of our lifestyle. There was no clear indication that gay couples would be accepted. All the wording on their materials talked about husbands and wives. Mothers and their children. Nothing about partners. Nothing about two women who are committed to each other, who are lost and confused, and full of fear.

Thankfully, we heard through the grapevine about the Mautner Project for Lesbians with Cancer. What luck! A place for lesbians to talk about cancer? Wahoo! I checked with my buddy the internet and found their address and phone number. We decided to pay them a visit.

The women at Mautner were very kind, and gave us information on their support group meetings. We were apprehensive, and nervous at first, as I'm sure most women are. But once there, we realized we were no different than the rest of the women there. At Mautner we found the comfort and support that we were desperately needing. What an amazing place. We quickly felt at home. I was happy to know that other partners felt the same frustrations, that I wasn't crazy, we were all doing our best.

One day, I put together my feelings on paper and decided to read it to the group during one of the meetings. I was amazed to find people with tears in their eyes after I finished reading. Then it hit me, we all felt this way. Some had different cancers, lived in different cities, some were partners, some were cancer patients, but we all had one thing in common: Cancer. I wasn't alone, and neither were they. It was a comforting realization.

There was a bitter/sweet feeling when a new person came to the group. One moment I would feel excited because I was meeting someone for the first time, making a new friend, but on the other hand, knowing that one other woman had cancer, one other woman was fearing death, and would possibly be facing it, filled me with sadness and anger.

That year, we attended the Mautner's Gala, Brunie with her beautiful bald head, me with my spiked heels and long gown. My foo foo outfit as she called it. We had a great time. When someone on stage asked for the cancer survivors to stand so that we could honor them, I cried and cried, and even now, as I remember it, I get choked up. Brunie was in a new category. A cancer survivor. A cancer patient. Cancer. Then they asked the partners to stand up so that we could be honored too, and it was a beautiful moment. But when they asked for a moment of silence to honor and remember those who couldn't be there because of cancer, I lost it. I wished, and still hope, that I will never have to know what that will feel like. I cried for those partners out there who had lost someone to cancer. For Mary-Helen Mautner's partner.

Now, one year later, Brunie's cancer sometimes is a faded memory, until we hear about a new drug on the market, or read about someone else who has died because of it, then reality smacks us right in the face and we fear all over again. We decided to become volunteers for Mautner. After all they did for us, it was the least we could do. Being co-chairs for this year's Gala was an honor. It was an honor to work alongside such wonderful and caring people who give freely of their time to help women like us where we were last year.

Would I be the one this year to ask for the recognition of cancer survivors, of partners? Would I ask for the moment of silence? How could I not. It is a part of my everyday life.

Brunie continues to exercise, and take her vitamins, and we continue to eat healthfully. Her hair grew back more beautiful and curlier than ever. It's hard to complain now about bad hair days after seeing her with no hair days once. We now attend church regularly because we also found a new family and set of friends there. It's our soul food. We go for walks, and pay attention to the sound of leaves rustling, or the trees moving in the wind. We now know that mockingbirds, European starlings, sparrows, cardinals, blue jays, crows, mourning doves and an occasional woodpecker and goldfinch visit our backyard. We know what days the neighborhood men gather to play soccer behind our house. Swimming feels different now, freeing in a sense. We smile at the sight of a happy child, and hold each other and cry when we hear disheartening news on TV. We can most likely remember the way the sky looked on any given day, and don't complain when it rains. It feels good, the water on our skin. If it's hot, that feels nice too. All those feelings remind us we are alive.

When I think about what that pink ribbon stands for, I realize I have a love/hate relationship with cancer. I love it for all the beauty it has brought our lives, how it has changed our perspective. We truly value the most simple, joyful moments we spend with each other and in the company of others. I love it for the sweetness it has put in each of our hearts, for the way it has caused us to embrace life and honor God, honor our friends, honor our jobs. We had so much before, and never even stopped to be thankful. Now, we can't stop thanking. I hate it for the pain it caused us. I hate it for the fear it still fills us with when Brunie thinks she is sick, or when I explore her breasts each month, even when I explore mine. I hate it for the millions of lives it claims each year. I hate it for not being clear about why it happens.

I look at the pink ribbon and I see a loop, a reminder of the roller coaster of emotions that we have felt, with no clear beginning, and no clear end. That's cancer for you. I know that it's tied around my heart forever, with love and hate traveling through it all at once. Cancer is engraved in me.

I stare at her a lot now, a lot more than before, and just love her. I love to know that we have one more day to enjoy each other's company. I touch her soft curls and caress her eyebrows, and never forget when they weren't there.

As I looked out into the audience the other night, standing in front of the microphone in another foo foo outfit, I held my partner real tight because she's alive, and so am I, and her skin against mine feels real nice, like the sun and the rain do. It reminded me how alive we are, no matter what is happening to our physical body. When I was honoring the cancer survivors, the partners, the lost loved ones, I said it with every bit of love and truth that is in me because I truly understand the impact cancer has on our lives. I don't know how my voice sounded, I don't know really how I looked, but I do know that my heart was in it, ribbon and all.

# and the floods came

*Victoria A. Brownworth*

1.

on the thirteenth day of the flooding
allen ginsberg died
harpies of a long tempestuous life/feasting on his liver
he wrote poem after poem on his death bed
imagining all the flesh that became words
over one or another decade
surrounded by friends/old lovers/candles/books/chanting
until his heart gave out
chanting the kaddish of a life

*lived*

as shadows bend over the body/the voice of a beat generation
rises up like bread
from that unleavened pallet

all the words that flowed from his heart and mind
onto the page/into teenage souls inspired to face
adulthood     a legacy: *gay*
leaves of grass/*bossa nova*/censorship/*shiva*


2.

in the heartland/howl/cattle founder
on the tundrad shores of the red river
titanic chunks of ice crash along the levees
slam into trees/houses/barns/animals
an entire hog farm swallowed into the vortex
of rushing water/ thick with ice
in a whiteout 18 miles outside fargo, north dakota
where allen ginsberg never read a poem

up river     *flash*     aurora borealis out of season
near grand forks the power fails
breech birth in blizzard isolation
rends the night like ice cracking across the river crested
38 feet above flood stage and frozen at ten below zero
the mother howls/fears death in this stark blue-white world
will her child die?  or: be
one of the best minds of his generation
or a hog farmer/cattle rancher/still homesteading
well past the millennium strike
or a pedophile/stalker/serial killer/dead at 20 in a hail
of gunfire louder than the winds that rip power lines/shear
the lights from this chill birth night

*roar*

the words form/nonlinear/a blank verse of despair:

how can she travel through these hours till dawn
till bright blue sky blends with sunlight
belying the floods to come/water breaking
an episiotomy tear through the dike of sandbags
hand-filled by every farmer within the county
soon: an island born of this farm as the baby lies
pale blue howling at his mother's side


3.

on the seventeenth day of the flooding
laura nyro died
held tight
by one lover/one child/one sheaf of poems turned to song
seclusion: they'd forgotten the smoldering coal black eyes/
the thick wave of hair black and enveloping as chador
and a voice/a vortex of octaves as piano music crested
up and over the seventh floor walkup east side fire escape
flooding down to the ashcan kickball junkie street below

residuals: as others took her words/her notes/but not her
onto the airwaves/into the mainstream/leaving her stranded
on the shoreline of notoriety/bled of the sluicing words
that poured down one torrent after another
a thunderous flood of poetry

left: with one lover/one child/one thick sheaf of poems
turned to songs
as death approached/a shadow stranger her words created
this one creeping along in the body's dark night
through the pliant soft tissue/the womb
from which the child but not the poems came
the fecund lining: she had already birthed so much

no levee could keep this pain at bay
death smug and small/a flesh eater gnawing away
through
tiny dam breaks: hollowing the black eyes/
tearing the hair in handful after handful/and finally
silencing the voice/staunching the coursing heart/blood/beat
of words/of music/of deep smoky sound that howled
through the souls of so many women


4.

on the twenty-first day of the flooding
we are left/sitting *shiva* behind the cracking levee
the mouldering banks of sand and dirt
the tiny efforts of men and women
to hold back the fatal cascade/the seductive surging rush
the lethal red river
we are left: to staunch the flood/to blot the landscape
with our tortured cries
our unanswered prayers
our devastation  our last hope


we know our dead: the bloated bodies of cattle lain waste
along the hardened drifts of snow/the convex torsoes of deer
eviscerated by wind beneath the tattered bales of hay
fallen near the abandoned salt licks
the last six piglets frozen solid in a cake of icy mud
ten feet from the barn door and their dead mother
the ghosts of houses rise out of the mud-smudged whiteness
siloes stand like funerary sculptures on the decimated
farmland

we have lived here for generations

our voices have echoed through the vast plains
our words lent shape to the unfettered veldt
our lives delineated the landscape
our world is hard work/no-nonsense/dawn-to-dusk
we have faced the elements together
the canadian blast/the arctic wind/the blizzard months
we have held ourselves in check
we have held the river back
we have held on

we have been our own poetry

5.

what do we do when the dam shatters
when words fail and floods flash like wildfire through
our homes     our villages     our world
these are the words of emergency
the best minds of our generation
they bulk us up like levees
hold back the flood crest of despair until it can
subside/evaporate     diminish another season of flooding

recovery is slow from these acts of God
slaking thirst in a world suffused by tainted water
slogging through mud/peeling back the mildewed wallpaper
of a life
rending our garments through the pain of our many losses
they leave us words to cry in the midst of bleakness
the howl/the kaddish
the best minds of one generation or another
the best words
poems delivered from a death bed

*and the floods came*

from the death throes
the final lyrics left behind
a rosetta stone to decipher our loss
a canticle for our dead
a hymn for our future
an epitaph to hope


6.

those words, those words
the very last tones uttered before the floods came
the first sound we can cry out as we move forward into
the wet night soaked through with tears
on the shore of the red river
in the heartland    in America
as we watch our lives subside
again


Note:
The worst flooding ever to hit the Midwest occurred in late winter 1997, after the coldest and most blizzard-ridden winter in a century. During the time that the rivers continued to rise, poet Allen Ginsberg died of liver cancer and songwriter Laura Nyro died of ovarian cancer. Ginsberg was the most famous of the beat poets of the fifties; his work—especially *Howl*—altered the course of American poetry. Ginsberg was the first outspoken gay poet in America since Walt Whitman. Nyro's songs were chart-toppers throughout the seventies and eighties but usually as covers recorded by other artists—including the Fifth Dimension and Barbra Streisand. Nyro's smoky, languid musical style combined jazz and torch singing; her queer lyrics attracted a large lesbian audience.

# HEALTH INSURANCE: Getting Coverage for the Treatment You Need

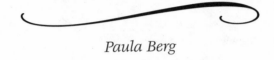

*Paula Berg*

THE UNITED STATES IS THE ONLY industrialized country in the world that does not provide all of its citizens with access to health care. As a result, the availability of medical care in the United States depends on whether people can afford to purchase coverage for themselves, whether they are covered by a group policy offered by an employer or union, or whether they qualify for coverage under a public program, such as Medicaid or Medicare. Approximately forty-three million Americans—nearly one in six people—lack any type of health insurance whatsoever. Despite the economic boom of recent years, the ranks of the uninsured increases by one hundred thousand people every month.

People who have health insurance are often subject to a variety of limitations on their coverage. For example, gay men and lesbians are generally excluded from coverage under their partner's plan unless it covers domestic partners. Health maintenance organizations (HMOs) usually restrict enrollees to particular "in-network" doctors and hospitals, require referrals for specialty care and require approvals for surgery and other expensive treatments and procedures. The insured are also subject to increasing out-of-pocket expenses because of rising deductibles, coinsurance payments, caps and restrictions on prescription drug coverage. In addition, many lesbians are excluded from coverage under their partner's plan because it does not cover domestic partners.

Although the U.S. health care system arguably shortchanges everyone, its failings are most dramatically experienced by people with a serious or chronic illness, such as cancer. Too often a cancer diagnosis precipitates two battles: one against the illness and the other against an insurance company or HMO. This chapter provides an overview of the laws that protect your right to health care and restrict the ability of insurers and HMOs to deny necessary care to people with cancer. It is intended as a practical guide to help you get the cancer care you want and deserve from the health care providers and hospitals of your choice.

*Private Health Insurance*

From an economic standpoint, those people with serious illnesses are considered undesirable by insurance companies and managed care organizations (MCOs). To exclude these individuals from coverage, insurers have used various practices to deny coverage outright or severely limit its scope. Fortunately, federal and state laws now prohibit many of the practices that have been used by insurance companies to discriminate on the basis of a person's illness or medical history. In 1996, Congress enacted the Health Insurance Portability and Accountability Act (HIPAA), which bars insurance companies and HMOs from denying enrollment to an applicant because of her health status, medical condition or medical history. HIPAA also prohibits insurers from refusing to renew or continue coverage because of an insured's health. Thus your application for health insurance coverage as an individual or as a member of a group cannot be rejected, and your coverage cannot be terminated, because you have cancer.

HIPAA also restricts the use of preexisting condition exclusions, which deny insurance coverage for a medical condition that existed before an applicant's enrollment. Preexisting condition exclusions force people with cancer to remain in their jobs because they fear losing coverage for cancer care under a new employer's health plan. Although preexisting condition exclusions remain legal under HIPAA, the law places limits on their applicability.[1] Under HIPAA, an insurer may impose a preexisting condition limitation only for conditions for which medical advice, diagnosis, care or treatment was recommended or received within a six-month period preceding the enrollment date. Thus, if you get a new job, were diagnosed with cancer more than six months before starting that job and did not receive any cancer care during this period, you cannot be subject to a preexisting condition exclusion for cancer care in the future. In addition, a genetic predisposition for cancer cannot be the basis for a preexisting condition exclusion.

Preexisting condition exclusions may only extend for twelve months. Moreover, if an applicant for individual or group coverage was covered within sixty-two days of applying for coverage under a new policy, she must be given credit for the period covered under the previous plan. Thus, if you work at a job for eight months and then change jobs, your new employer's plan must give you credit for the eight months that you were covered under your former employer's plan. Under the new plan individuals can be denied coverage for cancer care for only four months. If you were covered by your former employer's plan for more than one year, you may not be subject to any preexisting condition exclusion, as long as you apply for coverage within sixty-two days.

Applicants who do not obtain coverage under a new plan within sixty-two days of losing coverage under their old plan may be subject to the full twelve-month preexisting condition exclusion permitted by HIPAA.[2] Given this rule, if you are covered under an employer's plan and want to leave your job, and there is any chance that you may not be covered under a new policy within sixty-two days, you should keep your current coverage by paying for it yourself. A federal law called COBRA requires that employees who leave a job that provides health insurance must be offered the option of continuing their coverage for up to eighteen months by paying the cost of the premiums themselves. By continuing your coverage under COBRA, you will be assured of meeting HIPAA's sixty-two-day rule and having any preexisting condition exclusion in your new employer's plan reduced by the time you were covered under your prior plan.[3]

Although HIPAA prohibits some practices that make health insurance inaccessible to people with cancer and other serious illnesses, it has one huge shortcoming: It does not prohibit insurers from setting higher premiums because of a person's health status or medical history. Thus, although an insurer that does not want to continue covering an insured person with cancer can no longer terminate coverage, it can increase the premium and thereby effectively make coverage unaffordable and unavailable. While this practice, called "experience rating," does not violate federal law, some states, such as New York, have laws that prohibit premium rate setting on the basis of a person's or group's claims history.

## Publicly Financed Coverage

If you are not covered by a group insurance plan and cannot afford to purchase individual coverage for yourself, you may qualify for coverage under a public program. Medicaid is a federal-state cooperative program that provides medical coverage for certain low-income persons. It is important to understand, however, that Medicaid does not provide coverage to all poor persons. Instead, eligibility for Medicaid depends upon being poor *and* fitting into one of a number of categories defined by law.[4] Individuals who are eligible for Medicaid receive coverage for inpatient hospital services, outpatient hospital services, laboratory and x-ray services, skilled nursing facilities and physicians' services. In addition, most states provide additional benefits to Medicaid beneficiaries, such as coverage for prescription drugs, home health care and nursing home care.

Most of Medicaid's eligibility categories exclude many lesbians because they apply to families with children, pregnant women and children under nineteen. The categories that apply to low-income adults without children are limited. Many states offer coverage to the "medically needy," which applies to individuals who have high medical costs but do not qualify for Medicaid under another category. Under this program individuals must "spend down" any income or resources in excess of Medicaid's limits on medical bills in order to establish eligibility. In addition, recipients of Supplemental Security Income (SSI), which provides income support to low-income disabled persons, are eligible for Medicaid.

Medicare is the other major federal health care program in the United States. Although it primarily covers the elderly, it also applies to individuals who have received Social Security disability payments for two years. Recipients of Medicare receive coverage for inpatient hospitalization, skilled nursing facilities, home health services and hospice care. Medicare also helps pay the costs of physician's services, outpatient hospital services, medical equipment and other health services and supplies other than prescription drugs.

Finally, many states have programs that offer medical coverage to low-income uninsured residents. Eligibility for these programs typically depends on a person's income and assets.

### Dealing With Managed Care Organizations

Approximately four of five Americans who have health insurance are covered by a managed care plan. The term *managed care* refers to several different organizational arrangements that include a system for financing and delivering health care to enrollees. The most common types of MCOs are HMOs, preferred provider organizations (PPOs) and point-of-service plans (POS). Although these organizations differ in some important respects, they share certain mechanisms that are designed to cut the cost of health care. These include gatekeeping and prior authorization functions performed by an enrollee's primary care physician or an administrative unit of the MCO itself. Other cost-cutting mechanisms include restrictions that are intended to encourage enrollees to receive treatment from particular physicians and hospitals that have contracted with the MCO to provide services to enrollees at a discount.

In recent years managed care has come under considerable criticism for placing cost concerns over the health care needs of enrollees. People with serious and chronic illnesses have been among the most vocal critics of managed care. Congress has not passed a patients' bill of rights. However, most states have laws that give MCO enrollees some rights and prohibit certain practices that make care difficult to obtain. While each state law is different, many share certain features that are described below.

Access to Specialists

Access to specialty care, which is of particular concern to people with cancer, has been a major source of conflict between MCOs and enrollees. In response to consumer complaints, many states have enacted provisions to make specialty care more accessible. For example, some states require that enrollees with life-threatening or disabling conditions be permitted to designate a specialist as their primary care provider. Some states also require that enrollees who need ongoing care from a specialist receive a standing referral. These provisions eliminate the requirement that an enrollee obtain a referral from her primary care physician every time she needs to see a specialist.

If an MCO does not have an in-network health care provider with the appropriate training and experience to meet the health care needs of an enrollee, some states require that the enrollee be referred to an appropriate out-of-network specialist at no extra cost. If the cancer care centers within your MCO's network do not specialize in treating the particular type of cancer or tumor that you have, you should try to get a letter from your primary care physician or your in-network specialist that states this and a referral to an appropriate out-of-network provider or institution. Such a letter may persuade your MCO to authorize out-of-network specialty care in the first instance or, if it is initially denied, to reverse this decision upon review.

### Mandated Benefits

Many states mandate that MCOs provide all enrollees with certain benefits. For example, a number of states require that MCOs cover reconstructive surgery after a mastectomy and prohibit MCOs from unduly limiting the length of time that a woman can receive inpatient care after having a mastectomy. Some states mandate coverage for breast cancer screening and certain expensive cancer treatments, such as high-dose chemotherapy with autologous bone marrow transplantation and stem cell transplantation for the treatment of breast cancer. Many states prohibit MCOs from requiring prior authorization for certain types of treatment. For example, some states bar MCOs from requiring an approval for emergency care, as long as the enrollee has a reasonable belief that she needs to go to an emergency room. Some states also limit the time that an MCO can take in determining whether to preauthorize treatment that has been requested or recommended.

### Grievance Procedures

Most states require MCOs to set up a grievance or appeals process for enrollees to challenge denials of care and other adverse decisions. Some laws spell out the process that the MCO must follow in conducting an internal review and require that enrollees have the right to appeal a decision to an outside reviewer, such as the state's insurance commissioner or an independent panel. The question of whether enrollees have the right to obtain damages from a court that arise from an MCO's denial of treatment is in considerable flux. Some states have laws that bar this type of lawsuit. Some courts have held that ERISA, a federal law that regulates employment-related benefits, prevents enrollees who receive coverage through their employer from seeking damages for an MCO's denial of care. However, this trend may be changing. Recently, several courts permitted cases challenging treatment-related decisions by MCOs to proceed despite ERISA. In addition, a few states have passed laws that specifically give enrollees the right to sue if their MCO denied, delayed or modified treatment.

ACCESS TO EXPERIMENTAL AND ALTERNATIVE TREATMENTS

People with cancer may seek experimental treatments if standard therapies are ineffective. An experimental treatment may be offered as part of a clinical trial conducted by a hospital, or it may be prescribed by a physician because of promising reports in the medical literature. It is often difficult to obtain insurance coverage for experimental treatments. Health insurance contracts typically state that coverage for experimental treatments is excluded. Recently, some MCOs voluntarily agreed to pay some of the costs associated with clinical trials. A number of states now have laws that restrict the right of insurers and MCOs to deny coverage for experimental treatments.

For example, Rhode Island, which has the broadest of these laws, requires insurers and MCOs to cover "new cancer therapies" that are provided as part of an approved clinical trial to appropriate patients for whom there is no superior traditional treatment. South Carolina requires coverage for cancer drugs if their use is supported by the medical literature. Florida, New Jersey and Tennessee mandate coverage for particular cancer treatments—specifically, high-dose chemotherapy, bone marrow transplants and stem cell transplants— irrespective of the type of cancer that is being treated. Massachusetts, Minnesota, Missouri, New Hampshire and Virginia require coverage for certain experimental treatments for breast cancer. Georgia's law covers experimental treatments for breast cancer and Hodgkin's disease.

People whose needs fit within the boundaries of their state's law, as well as those who live in states that do not have such laws, are likely to have their initial request for an experimental therapy denied by their MCO or insurance company. Enrollees in managed care plans are generally required to initially challenge a denial of coverage through an internal review process. Often this review process must be expedited if an enrollee has a terminal condition. In addition, some states require that MCOs also offer an external review process.

If you lose an appeal to your HMO, you can challenge the decision in court. However, this process can be quite protracted and as a result, highly problematic if you need immediate treatment. Moreover, court decisions in this area have been quite inconsistent. Lawsuits challenging the denial of coverage for experimental treatments focus on the definition of this term in the insurance contract. If the definition is unambiguous, it will be enforced by the court. However, if the definition is ambiguous (which it usually is) courts will consider whether the therapy has the support of the medical community, whether its use is intended to help the patient or further research, and whether the denial of coverage was based merely on the insurer's economic self-interest or on genuine uncertainty about the treatment's efficacy.

People with cancer often look to alternative and complementary medicine to aid in the treatment of cancer and to alleviate some of the side effects of standard treatments. Some states require coverage for particular types of alternative therapy, such as chiropractic treatment. Also, MCOs are increasingly choosing to offer coverage for some alternative therapies, such as acupuncture and nutritional therapy. Usually, however, coverage is conditioned upon the enrollee's obtaining a referral from a primary care physician or choosing an in-network alternative provider. Some MCOs also offer riders to their standard contract that provide enhanced coverage for alternative and complementary therapies.

Notes:
1. Some states have laws that are even more restrictive of preexisting condition exclusions than HIPAA.
2. Under HIPAA any waiting period for coverage under a group plan may not be taken into account in determining whether a break in creditable coverage has occurred. Thus the key date for measuring the sixty-two-day continuous coverage requirement is the date of employment by the new employer, not the date upon which health insurance coverage under the new employer's plan actually takes effect.
3. Time spent covered under COBRA must also be deducted from a twelve-month preexisting condition exclusion.
4. States determine Medicaid's eligibility criteria. Therefore, it is necessary to contact your state's department of social services to find out whether you are eligible.

# AGAINST ELEGIES
*for Catherine Arthur and Melvin Dixon*

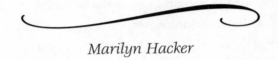

*Marilyn Hacker*

James has cancer. Catherine has cancer.
Melvin has AIDS.
Whom will I call, and get no answer?
My old friends, my new friends who are old,
or older, sixty, seventy, take pills
with meals or after dinner. Arthritis
scourges them. But irremediable night is
farther away from them; they seem to hold
it at bay better than the young-middle-aged
whom something, or another something, kills
before the chapter's finished, the play staged.
The curtains stay down when the light fades.

Morose, unanswerable, the list
of thirty- and forty-year-old suicides
(friends' lovers, friends' daughters) insists

in its lengthening: something's wrong.
The sixty-five-year-olds are splendid, vying
with each other in work hours and wit.
They bring their generosity along,
setting the tone, or not giving a shit.
How well, or how eccentrically, they dress!
Their anecdotes are to the point, or wide
enough to make room for discrepancies.
But their children are dying.

Natalie died by gas in Montpeyroux.
In San Francisco, Ralph died
of lung cancer, AIDS years later, Lew
wrote to me. Lew, who, at forty-five,
expected to be dead of drink, who, ten
years on, wasn't, instead, survived
a gentle, bright, impatient younger man.
(Cliché: he falls in love with younger men.)
Natalie's father came, and Natalie,
as if she never had been there, was gone.
Michèle closed up their house (where she
was born). She shrouded every glass inside

—mirrors, photographs—with sheets, as Jews
do, though she's not a Jew.
James knows, he thinks, as much as he wants to.
He hasn't seen a doctor since November.
They made the diagnosis in July.
Catherine is back in radiotherapy.
Her schoolboy haircut, prematurely gray,
now frames a face aging with other numbers:
"stage two," "stage three" mean more than "fifty-one"
and mean, precisely, nothing, which is why
she stares at nothing: lawn chair, stone,
bird, leaf; brusquely turns off the news.

I hope they will be sixty in ten years
and know I used their names
as flares in a polluted atmosphere,
as private reasons where reason obtains
no quarter. Children in the streets
still die in grandfathers' good wars.
Pregnant women with AIDS, schoolgirls, crack whores,
die faster than men do, in more pain,
are more likely than men to die alone.
And our statistics, on the day I meet
the lump in my breast, you phone
the doctor to see if your test results came?

The earth-black woman in the bed beside
Lidia on the AIDS floor—deaf, and blind:
I want to know if, no, how, she died.
The husband, who'd stopped visiting, returned?
He brought the little boy, those nursery-
school smiles taped on the walls?  She traced
her name on Lidia's face
when one of them needed something. She learned
some Braille that week. Most of the time, she slept.
Nobody knew the baby's HIV
status. Sleeping, awake, she wept.
And I left her name behind.

And Lidia, where's she
who got her act so clean
of rum and Salem Filters and cocaine
after her passing husband passed it on?
As soon as she knew
she phoned and told her mother she had AIDS
but no, she wouldn't come back to San Juan.
Sipping *café con leche* with dessert,
in a blue robe, thick hair in braids,

she beamed: her life was on the right
track, now. But the cysts hurt
too much to sleep through the night.

No one was promised a shapely life
ending in·a tutelary vision.
No one was promised: if
you're a genuinely irreplaceable
grandmother or editor
you will not need to be replaced.
When I die, the death I face
will more than likely be illogical:
Alzheimer's or a milk truck: the absurd.
The Talmud teaches we become impure
when we die, profane dirt, once the word
that spoke this life in us has been withdrawn,

the letter taken from the envelope.
If we believe the letter will be read,
some curiosity, some hope
come with knowing that we die.
But this was another century
in which we made death humanly obscene:
Soweto  El Salvador  Kurdistan
Armenia  Shatila  Baghdad  Hanoi
Auschwitz  Each one, unique as our lives are,
taints what's left with complicity,
makes everyone living a survivor
who will, or won't bear witness for the dead.

I can only bear witness for my own
dead and dying, whom I've often failed:
unanswered letters, unattempted phone
calls, against these fictions. A fiction winds
her watch in sunlight, cancer ticking bone

to shards. A fiction looks
at proofs of a too-hastily finished book
that may be published before he goes blind.
The old, who tell good stories, half expect
that what's written in their chromosomes
will come true, that history won't interject
a virus or a siren or a sealed
train to where age is irrelevant.
The old rebbetzin at Ravensbrück
died in the most wrong place, at the wrong time.
What do the young know different?
No partisans are waiting in the woods
to welcome them. Siblings who stayed home
count down doom. Revolution became
a dinner party in a fast-food chain,
a vendetta for an abscessed crime,
a hard-on market for consumer goods.
A living man reads a dead woman's book.
She wrote it; then, he knows, she was turned in.

For every partisan
there are a million gratuitous
deaths from hunger, all-American
mass murders, small wars,
the old diseases and the new.
Who dies well? The privilege
of asking doesn't have to do with age.
For most of us
no question what our deaths, our lives, mean.
At the end, Catherine will know what she knew,
and James will, and Melvin,
and I, in no one's stories, as we are.

# Living with Cancer

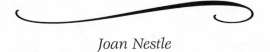

*Joan Nestle*

*Early Words*
*January 15, 1997*

I haven't been able to write a word since I was told I have stage-two colon cancer in 1996. All of it—the bleeding, the tests, the operation, the chemo, the fissure that would not heal and the doctors who did everything so fast and did not listen to me—all embody everything I detest, including my own body. Embody. I embody disease and disavowal, blood and shit and body bound in pain. Everything tastes like acid now, like car batteries in my mouth. If ever words could bring me life, and they have, please, please do it now.

A memory: Bayside, Queens, 1952, in the housing development. My twelve-year-old body covered in welts, huge red platelets signifying the body's anger with penicillin. My mother had to go to work. I had pleaded with her to call a doctor, never a child's desire, but we didn't have the money and she didn't have the time. That morning when she saw the welts, she must have known that I needed help. She went to work, but the doctor did come. Did I call the doctor? Did my mother, from the confines of her bookkeeper's office?

Have I softened this memory? The young doctor came into our disheveled apartment. "Where is your mother? Does she often leave you like this?" he asked, as he poured baking powder into the bathtub, helping me lower my tormented body into the cooling bath. "You could have died from this." After the bath, he took me back to my bed and sprinkled the sheets with the same cooling powder. Perhaps he gave me medication to counter-effect the body's anger, I do not remember, but he gave me concern and relief; he gave me care. Another history we have, the history of those who cared for our bodies.

*January 23, 1997*
*In the midst of cancer.*

Riverside Park in New York City on an early evening in January, the night growing colder by the moment, walking Perry on the adventure I promised him and me. The curve of the bowl-shaped lawn running deep down to the playground—just a shadowy empty town now—the old trees, stark and adamant, surrounding us. We walk up to the plaza in front of the Civil War memorial—always a special place for me, the prow of a ship with a tattered flag whipping in the wind, the stone steps leading up to the marble mausoleum, the frozen-in-stone cannonballs passed on the way. I would sit on those steps on summer afternoons with Denver, her big body resting against me, her shaggy head turned straight ahead—she was the captain of my ship. Always I have adventured in little places, but the glow of freedom, Denver off her leash, Perry running free in the marbled night, choosing to sit with me, to return to my side—these were wonders. Now, tonight, I give this walk as my gift, for a few minutes Perry and I are adventurers in the night, the plaza all ours, a fifty-seven-year-old lesbian and her dog, a woman with cancer and her dog, the flag of no country straining in the wind, clinking its tether against the masthead of a white iron pole. Soon the cold seeps through my coat, and I turn us toward home. As we walk farther away from the park, the night growing darker, I am walking farther and farther from all I love.

I hate what is happening to me, I hate the pain, the numbness, the nausea, the cold, the chemo pills waiting for me like small bombs in the plastic bag. I hate it all.

*February 25, 1997*

"Cancer cells are immortal," said the article in the *New York Times*. "They grow forever in the laboratory." I sit looking at these words. I and so many others are the hosts to this indomitable life form, a cellular surge to move ahead, leaving us fragile in its wake. Every Tuesday night, I go to a Cancer Care support group, my CR group of the 1990s, seven women, none of us immortal. We come with our bodies scarred by surgeries and treatments, by insertions and removals, we come to tell what the week has brought us. Some speak of the small pleasures they do not want to lose, the warmth of sunlight, the excitement of a trip, the taste of food. We talk of night terrors and loss of lovers. While the cancer cells inside us glory in their dedication to life, we mark our survival by their death. Doctors call it a war; I do not yet know what to call it, this push and pull between a cell's minute and yet endless passion for life and my own organically larger but perhaps not as determined need to live.

I have always delighted in the richness of contradictions, but this one gives no pleasure, no surge of intellectual insight or emotional wisdom. I do not yet know how to come to terms with the cancer inside of me. The chemotherapy sickens every part of me, body and spirit.

I know I am supposed to be a fighter, a warrior against the intruders, but in these early words I cannot be. I have always wanted to write hope, to inscribe yearnings—the moments when the face turned to the sun. For now, however, I only have these words, but others, many others, many many others, have found syllables of defiance.

*Three Years Later*
*March 5, 2000*

Now I am angry, angry at the pollution of land, food and water by businesses and governments that do not care how many die from their way of making money. I am angry at the cancer business of hospital centers, drug cartels, doctors who sneer at managed health programs and managed health programs that do not reimburse doctors with a reasonable amount of money in a reasonable duration of time. I am angry at how mundane, how prolific this illness has become. I am angry at my own feelings of stigmatization, so reminiscent of how I felt in the late 1950s when I came out as a fem in the bars of

New York. Once again I feel the shame of inherent failure, of biological deformity. I want collective militant action; I want us, the scarred and the amputated, the seared and the surgically rearranged, to throw our bodies against their daily schedules of business as usual, to botch up the works, to turn this fragile flesh into a wall of No More.

## My Cancer Travels

This is now my battle: to win back from the specifics of medical treatment—from the outrage of an invaded body where hands I did not know touched parts of myself that I will never see. My own body, my own body so marked by the hands and lips of lovers, now so lonely in its fear. Touch my scar, knead my belly, don't be afraid of my cancer. Enter me the old way, not through the skin cut open, but because I am calling to you through the movement of my hips, the breath that pleads for your hand to touch the want of me. Heal me because you do not fear me, touch me because you do not fear the future. Cancer and sex. One I have and one I must have.

Notes:
"Early Words" was first published in the New York City Lesbian Health Fair Journal, May 3, 1997.
"My Cancer Travels" was first published in A Fragile Union: New and Selected Writings (San Francisco: Cleis Press, 1999).

# ROSE AND VIVIAN
## A Love Story

Lisa D. Williamson

SUCH NAIVETÉ AND INNOCENCE are usually reserved for fairy tales. Even Vivian Kasper herself, looking back, remembers her ingenuousness with a kind of mild wonder.

"Therein lies our kind of unusual thing," says seventy-three-year-old Vivian now, of the beginning of her thirty-four-year relationship with Rosemarie Nixon. "I never even knew another lesbian. Rosie was the only one, was the first one."

Vivian was in her twenties, living with her mother and her sister, when she was first introduced to Rosie in 1950. She was not unworldly; as a design engineer for the telephone company in Baltimore, she helped develop telephone systems for businesses throughout Maryland. Although Vivian's living arrangements were perhaps sheltered—she never saw the need to waste money on a place of her own and was content to live with her mother and sister— Vivian led an active life. In addition to her career, she belonged to bowling leagues. And that's how she met Rosie. A friend introduced the two. They ended up bowling on the same team, and after little more than a year, Vivian and Rosie moved in together.

They were very nearly the same age. Vivian was born on Christmas Day in 1927, Rosie three weeks later on January 18. "She tortured me about those three weeks," Vivian laughs now, "by saying I was older than she was." Vivian and Rosie had a lot of laughs together. As many single women were advised, Rosie appeared in the phone book as R. M. Nixon.

"That was a fun set of initials to have," Vivian says. "But getting telephone calls at two o'clock in the morning for Tricky Dick was not fun."

Although Vivian was naive about moving in with Rosie, her old friend from the bowling league soon put her to rights. "The friend that introduced me to Rose told me that I was gross, and that she couldn't stand me," remembers Vivian now. "I said, 'Why?' She said, 'The terrible things you do.' I don't even know what I do. I didn't know anything. She just said that's it. She didn't want to talk to me; she didn't want to see me. It was like a group of people all involved in the league, and word got out to all of them very rapidly. It wasn't that anybody was unkind, it just seemed like people stopped talking when we came in. Subjects changed very fast, and things like that. It got uncomfortable, so we just stopped going. We didn't know anybody."

Even though Vivian and Rose would spend a long, satisfying life together, it was an isolated life. Gone was the recreation. Vivian's mother and sister did not speak to the two for five years. Although both worked—Vivian at the telephone company, and Rose as an assistant manager for Coke—neither was particularly wrapped up in company social life. Further, where Vivian had little past to speak of, Rose did not talk about her own past. Vivian knew Rose had been in prior relationships, but they were not discussed. "We never talked about it," says Vivian. "The past was over. Nothing that happened had anything to do with us. We were living today and in the future." For thirty-four years, this philosophy worked. Rose had her mother and a couple of aunts she was close with, and after a five-year hiatus, Vivian's mother and sister resumed speaking with Vivian. In fact, Rose and Vivian's mother became extremely close. But that was the extent of Vivian and Rose's universe. Shunned by the straight community, they were—at least Vivian was—unaware that there was a whole other world. Things were fine, until Rose became sick.

It all began right after Christmas, just before Rose turned fifty-seven.

"She said she was feeling badly and wanted to go to the doctor," recalls Vivian. "She just thought she was ill. She went to the doctor and they thought she might have pneumonia. They gave her medication for a week and she didn't respond in any way, so they sent her for a breathing test. That led to sending her for a biopsy."

The results were not good. It was lung cancer, and the treatment was radiation. Rose and Vivian were hopeful, however; the doctor, the head of oncology at one of the better hospitals in the Baltimore area, was very positive. In fact, Rose's biggest worry was not about herself, but about her Aunt Alice, who was in a nursing home. Rose was in the habit of visiting Alice daily, and made Vivian promise to carry on this practice if anything happened. Vivian was not overly alarmed about Rose's condition at this point either.

"I couldn't really believe it," she remembers. "You know those things happen, but they never happen to anybody you know or anybody you care about." Rose had had a previous scare, about five years earlier. At this time both she and Vivian were smokers. Rose had developed laryngitis and gone to a doctor, who had asked her if she smoked.

"He told her to stop it as of right now, don't do it again," recollects Vivian. "And she did." But Rose's willpower didn't last long. As soon as she got a clean bill of health, she resumed smoking.

"She was a very determined woman," Vivian adds. "When she wanted to diet, you could not tempt her with anything in this world. But she couldn't give up smoking. I know she wanted to, but she couldn't. Even when she got sick [the second time], she couldn't give it up." By the time of her lung cancer diagnosis, Rose was completely hooked. She even asked Vivian to smuggle in cigarettes when she had to stay in the hospital. "I said, 'Rose, I can't do that. You know I can't do that,'" Vivian recalls. "Well, she cried. And I cried. And we knew about cancer, and I thought, 'What the hell?' And I went and brought her two packs of cigarettes. But I said, 'Please don't ever ask me to do this again.' She did smoke them, though."

By this time Rose and Vivian had become even more isolated socially. Rose's mother had died, as had Vivian's. Both Vivian and Rose had retired early, and they had no close friends. Vivian's sister was living by herself in an apartment, so she moved into their house to help out. Because of the radiation, Rose was in a lot of pain, so the doctor sent her to a pain management clinic. Vivian and her sister needed to help Rose get to the treatments. "I never did understand [the pain management clinic]. I think what they tried to do is literally torture you, so you wouldn't remember your pain," says Vivian. "They put her on bicycles to pedal. They did all kinds of things at this pain management clinic. She would go there, and it was different kinds of exercise. Then they would do a kind of a heat treatment. She said that was good; the rest of it, she said, was just agony. We used to go to radiation therapy every day, Monday through Friday. Then from there, three times a week, we went over to the pain management clinic."

Vivian would drive to these appointments, and while she was finding a place to park, her sister would help Rose into the clinic and on into the hospital. "I drove her to the treatments, but at first I wouldn't go in with her," remembers Vivian. "My sister would go in with her. I would wait out in the waiting room. I just couldn't go in and see what they were doing to her. I never did go in when they gave her the radiation. I just couldn't walk in that room."

Things seemed to be getting better, however. The mass in Rose's lung began to decrease. Then all of a sudden, three months into treatment, Vivian received a phone call from the doctor. "He said the cancer showed up in the other lung, and there's nothing we can do now. No more treatment, no more nothing."

Vivian received this news on her own and had to break it to Rosie, who ended up being the stronger emotionally of the two. In retrospect, Vivian thinks that Rosie suspected the worst all along. "I was just crying," Vivian recalls. "She was better than me. I think maybe in the dark of night, when you're not sleeping, things occur to you."

Rose's insurance covered all the costs, and she had transferred power of attorney to Vivian. From these perspectives, there were no problems. No one ever excluded Vivian from Rose's treatment; she was never made to feel unwelcome. Rather, their lifelong isolation became the bigger problem. Neither Vivian nor Rose had much outside support, other than Vivian's sister. A hospice chaplain and nurses and aides would visit the house, but there were no personal friends.

After Rose's second diagnosis, things went downhill rapidly. She was given morphine for her pain, and had a severe reaction to it. From that point on, for the last six or seven weeks, she could eat nothing. "They tried everything under the sun," recalls Vivian. "I clearly remember having to go to the drugstore, and the prescription was for methadone. Driving home, I was scared to death, knowing I had methadone. They hoped it was something they could give her to help quell the nausea. It didn't."

Rose died on July 24, six months from the date of her first diagnosis. Her death, of course, left Vivian even more alone. But neither regretted their life and those final months together. Even toward the end, they were completely wrapped up in each other. "We talked at length about things, still looking with hope that there was a future," says Vivian. "At that point, we knew there wasn't any future, but we did live together. We had a beautiful life together, just the two of us. We didn't have any more friends; we just did things together. All the time; we were never, ever apart."

The one thing that was missing, however, was an outside life. Vivian had been completely unaware of a larger lesbian community, and Rose had never mentioned one. "The thing that bothers me the most is the deep regret that I have that I didn't know any of this existed, so that Rose and I could have been such a part of it," Vivian adds now. "I still wonder about that, why she never talked about anything. But we never talked about the past. I knew she was living with someone when I [met] her. They broke up, and that's how we got together. But we never talked about it."

Fortunately, the fairy tale life that Rose and Vivian had enjoyed did not end with Rose's death. Gradually, Vivian began to become aware of an entire lesbian subculture that had been denied her during Rose's life. She made a friend—"the first friend that I made [after Rosie's death]"—who ran a bookstore in Washington, D. C. Through this friend she met more women and was invited to a gay pride parade. These experiences slowly introduced Vivian to a world she had never before realized existed.

Vivian volunteered to help the Mautner Project for Lesbians with Cancer and has attended the organization's gala since 1997. She is on the staff of the *Baltimore Women's Times*, helping publish their local calendar. She visits with newfound friends and goes to book signings and concerts.

"I guess I have almost two kinds of situations," Vivian notes. "Where I live, it's a gated community. I'm on the board of directors. I don't know if they know [I'm a lesbian]. I've never told them. They know I'm a casual dresser—I wear pants a lot—but no one has ever said anything to me [about being a lesbian]. I have never said anything to anyone. Then I have this other life, where I have a lot of friends who I know are lesbians, and who know I am."

Vivian loves the life she has carved out for herself and regrets not having known about these resources when she and Rose could have enjoyed them together. Still, the essence of their life together was not "lesbian" or "straight"—it was love.

"We were two people," she says. "It's funny. [My friend] said something, why I didn't know or didn't think about being a lesbian. I don't [think about] things like that. I was Vivian, who was in love with Rose, and Rose was in love with Vivian. We didn't call it any names. It was just us together."

# Permissions

"That Ribbon Around My Heart" by Olga Alvarado-Cofresi from *Zora's Journal*. Reprinted by permission of the author.

"Thanks for the Mammaries" by Alison Bechdel. Copyright © 1992. Reprinted by permission of the author.

"Vibrator Party" from *Lovers: Love and Sex Stories* by Tee A. Corinne. Reprinted by permission of the author.

"Murder at the Nightwood Bar" excerpted from *Murder at the Nightwood Bar* by Katherine Forrest. Reprinted by permission.

"A Scar I Did Not Want to Hide" by Jerilyn Goodman originally appeared in the March 24, 1994 issue of *Newsweek* magazine. Reprinted by permission of the author.

"Against Elegies", from WINTER NUMBERS by Marilyn Hacker. Copyright © 1994 by Marilyn Hacker. Used by permission of the author and W. W. Norton & Company, Inc.

"'A Private Little Hell': Selected Letters of Rachel Carson" excerpted from *A Darker Ribbon* by Ellen Leopold. Copyright © 1999 Ellen Leopold. Reprinted by permission of Beacon Press, Boston.

"A Burst of Light" from *A Burst of Light* by Audre Lorde. Copyright © 1988 by Audre Lorde. Reprinted by permission of Firebrand Books, Ithaca, New York.

"Self-Examination" (revised version) by Mona Oikawa. A version of "Self-Examination" was first published in *The Poetry of Sex: Lesbians Write the Erotic* edited by Tee Corinne. Austin, Texas: Edward-William Publishing Company, 1992. Reprinted by permission of the author.

"It's Not So Bad" and "Massage" from *Movement in Black* by Pat Parker. Copyright © 1999 by Pat Parker. Reprinted by permission of Firebrand Books, Ithaca, New York.

"Fitting Lesbians into Breast Cancer Activism: An Interview with Dr. Susan Love" by Paige Parvin originally appeared in the October 14, 1999 issue of *Southern Voice*, Atlanta's gay and lesbian newspaper. Reprinted by permission of *Southern Voice*.

"A Woman Dead in Her Forties", from THE FACT OF A DOORFRAME: Poems Selected and New, 1950–1984 by Adrienne Rich. Copyright © 1984 by Adrienne Rich. Copyright © 1975, 1978 by W. W. Norton & Company, Inc. Copyright © 1981 by Adrienne Rich. Used by permission of the author and W. W. Norton & Company, Inc.

# Acknowledgments

This book, doing triple duty as anthology, historical document and fundraiser, required a great deal of networking help from a range of people— too many to name here, but to all those involved, I trust you know how appreciative I am. In these times, when many have forgotten the importance of political activism, I am gratified to have had such warm response from so many women throughout the development of this project.

I would like to thank Nancy Bereano of Firebrand Books for her suggestions and support. From the inception of this project to its completion her advice was invaluable and I am not sure I would have undertaken this book without her encouragement and help. Nancy puts people and politics above the bottom line and in so doing provides a model for us all.

Deep appreciation to Diane DeKelb-Rittenhouse, student, friend and cancer survivor, who devoted myriad hours to cheerful and uncomplaining typing for this project when she could have been working on her own writing. Thanks to Tee A. Corinne for her love and support. Thanks also to Lisa D. Williamson and Joanne Dahme for their interviews; to Lynn Kanter and Paula Berg for their well-researched and essential pieces; to Deborah Peifer and Thea Spires; to Barbara Smith and Joan Nestle, vital activists; to Jerilyn Goodman, Julie Van Orden and Mona Oikawa; to Katherine V. Forrest; to Teya Schaffer, who shared her life with Jackie Winnow and carries Jackie's memory to another generation; to Sandra Butler who perpetuates the memory of Barbara Rosenblum; to Kelly Marbury and Vivian Kasper for sharing their stories; to Alison Bechdel, who keeps us laughing; to Sandra Steingraber, whose unflinching environmental activism mitigates my rage; to Marilyn Hacker, whose devotion to form inspires me; to Adrienne Rich, whose devotion to feminism inspires us all.

Thanks to Marian Hunstiger and Joan Drury of Spinster's Ink; Claire Reinertsen and Arlene Phalon of W. W. Norton & Co.; Allison Monro of Beacon Press; Midge Stocker of Third Side Press; Chris Crain, Joan Sherwood and Paige Parvin of *Southern Voice*.

For their continued generosity and dedication to women's lives, I am indebted to Joan Poole and Carolyn Phillips. For editorial suggestions and friendship, thanks to Charlotte Abbott and Roberto Friedman. Thanks to Story Clapp for her help and support. Thanks to Jennie Goldenberg, Theodore Brownworth, Leigh Love, Jane Shaw, Dr. Tish Fabens, the MSbians and the Living girls.

For her vital friendship and all those trips to Borders, thanks to Martha Peech. Thanks to Madelaine Gold for her friendship and generous help with this project.

Many thanks to Judith M. Redding for her editorial support and advice, her general commiseration on publishing issues and for thought-provoking conversation.

I am deeply grateful to Roberta L. Hacker, whose friendship and care have sustained me in the dark times when I did not think I would survive. As ever, I remain appreciative of my comrade in the life of the mind, Ruthann Robson, who consistently raises the intellectual bar.

For inspiring courage and fierceness, I am indebted to the late Audre Lorde. I shall never forget the night when I was twenty-five that we met and danced. Audre wrote the primer on how to live with cancer; when I met her, I never knew how much I would need her instruction.

Thanks to all the Seals, for coming through once again to support a vital lesbian issue, with special thanks to Faith Conlon, who perpetuates feminist publishing in a postfeminist era. Much appreciation to Jennie Goode for her equanimity in the face of editorial Sturm und Drang, for patience during those late night and weekend calls, for being a judicious editor and for her support of and devotion to lesbian politics. Thanks also to Alison Rogalsky and Anne Mathews for their careful efforts to ensure the accuracy of the reprinted pieces in this book; and to Amy Smith Bell for her thorough copyediting.

Finally, thanks to the Mautner Project for Lesbians with Cancer, and to executive director Kathleen DeBold, whose idea this book was, for their dedication to lesbians with cancer and their determination to save lesbian lives in the face of this epidemic. This book is for them and for all the women, like my late friend Shark La Bance, Audre, Laura Nyro, Barbara Deming, Rachel Carson and all those whose names we do not know, who did not survive being a lesbian with cancer in America.

# About the Contributors

Olga R. Alvarado-Cofresi grew up in Miami, Florida, and moved to Virginia in 1991. Since her move, she has worked in support positions ranging from legal secretary to marketing assistant to, most recently, senior staff secretary for a Department of Defense contractor. Writing has been a hobby of hers since childhood. She went for a number of years without writing anything, until her partner's breast cancer diagnosis. In search of an emotional outlet, she found comfort once again with pen and paper in hand. Since then, some of her poems and writings have been published in small magazines and newsletters. Alvarado-Cofresi lives in Virginia with her lifetime companion Brunie, and their daughter Luna. She is now a stay-at-home mom.

Alison Bechdel has been drawing the comic strip *Dykes To Watch Out For* since 1983. Nine collections of her award-winning cartoons, including the most recent *Post-Dykes To Watch Out For,* have been published by Firebrand Books. Her strip appears biweekly in seventy publications in the United States and Canada. She lives in Vermont.

Paula Berg is a health law professor at City University of New York Law School.

Sandra Butler authored the ground-breaking book *Conspiracy of Silence: The Trauma of Incest,* which has become a classic source and reference guide to the complex issues of incest. *Cancer in Two Voices,* written in collaboration with Barbara Rosenblum, was the winner of the Lambda Literary Award for Lesbian Non-Fiction in 1992. It is a personal document of living and dying, designed to make the private experience of terminal illness public, and therefore, political. Butler's trainings and seminars are attended by therapists, trainers, organizers and others interested in the relationship of personal growth to social change activism. In addition to her work in the field of child sexual assault and the politics of women's health, Butler is the co-director of the Institute for Feminist Training. In this capacity, she specializes in training, supervision and program consultation with individuals working in all forms of feminist psychological theory and practice, political organizing and cross-cultural work.

Rachel Carson founded the modern ecology movement, now known as environmentalism. Her groundbreaking book *Silent Spring* has become required reading in school curricula nationwide. Carson was diagnosed with breast cancer in 1960 and throughout her illness investigated the role of environmental issues in causing cancer, a role we now know to be significant.

Tee A. Corinne is a writer and artist whose books include *The Cunt Coloring Book, Courting Pleasure, The Sparkling Lavender Dust of Lust, Lovers:*

*Love and Sex Stories* and *Dreams of the Woman Who Loved Sex*. *Lambda Book Report* named her in its list of the fifty most influential lesbians and gay men of the 1980s. In 1997 she received the Women's Caucus for Art President's Award for service to women in the arts, and in 2000 she received the Abdill-Ellis Lifetime Achievement Award. According to *Completely Queer: The Gay and Lesbian Encyclopedia*, "Corinne is one of the most visible and accessible lesbian artists in the world."

Joanne Dahme has worked for the Philadelphia Water Department for eighteen years, most recently as General Manager of Public Affairs. Her fiction has appeared in numerous publications and anthologies, including *Night Bites: Vampire Tales by Women* and *Night Shade: Gothic Tales by Women*. Dahme is currently completing her second master's degree in the creative writing program at Temple University and is writing an historical novel set in Victorian Philadelphia. She lives in Roxborough, Pennsylvania with her husband and son.

Katherine V. Forrest is author and editor of twelve books, including seven Kate Delafield mysteries and the best-selling lesbian romance of all time, *Curious Wine*. She has won the Lambda Literary Award twice. Her most recent book is *Sleeping Bones: A Kate Delafield Mystery*. Forrest is currently working on a sequel to her classic novel *Daughters of a Coral Dawn*.

Madelaine Gold is an artist whose work has been exhibited in numerous group and one-woman shows. She has an MFA in painting from Platt Institute of Art and has been the recipient of numerous grants and awards including a Ford Foundation grant for painting. She has taught painting and design at the University of the Arts in Philadelphia for the past twenty-five years.

Jerilyn Goodman was diagnosed with breast cancer in 1993, at the age of forty-three, five years after she began telling her doctors about a suspicious thickening in her breast. She was fortunate to be living in Los Angeles at the time, where she encountered the very best of both American and Chinese medicine. With out lesbian Susan Love as her surgeon, Goodman was spared all those annoying questions about birth control. She is currently, and gratefully, alive and well and working in Washington, D.C., as press secretary to Congresswoman Tammy Baldwin, the first out lesbian in Congress.

Marilyn Hacker is the author of, most recently, *Winter Numbers* and *Selected Poems: 1965-1990*. She is also the author of *Presentation Piece*, a Lamont Poetry Selection and a National Book Award winner; *Love, Death and the Changing of the Seasons; Separations; Taking Notice; Assumptions;* and *Going Back to the River*. She is director of the masters program in creative writing and literature at the City College of New York and lives in New York City and Paris.

Roberta L. Hacker is the chief executive officer and executive director of Women in Transition, a feminist agency serving women who are experiencing domestic violence and/or substance abuse. Since 1988 she has provided leadership in organizing a coordinated citywide response to ending violence against women and children. Hacker currently serves as co-chair of the Philadelphia Family Violence Coordinating Council. She is also a core member of the Philadelphia Women's Death Review Team and is a member of the Board of Directors of the Pennsylvania Coalition Against Domestic Violence. In the past two decades Hacker has also served as the chief executive of Voyage House, Philadelphia's premiere agency for runaway and homeless youth, and as secretary for the National Network for Runaway and Homeless Youth. In 1984 she received the City of Philadelphia's Commission on Human Relations Human Rights Award for her work on behalf of women and children. From 1974 to 1985 she produced "Amazon Country," a one-hour weekly lesbian-feminist radio program on WXPN-FM.

Lynn Kanter wrote *The Mayor of Heaven*, a novel about a lesbian couple coping with breast cancer and loss. Her first novel, *On Lill Street*, was published in 1992, and her stories and essays have appeared in numerous anthologies. Kanter works for an anti-poverty organization in Washington, D.C.

Vivian Kasper worked for C&P Telephone in Baltimore, Maryland, as a design engineer and designed telephone systems for large and small businesses. She is currently retired and lives with her sister in Towson, Maryland. Kasper does volunteer work with a group of women that publishes the *Baltimore Women's Times* and is an avid reader. She and Rose were partners for over thirty years.

Ellen Leopold wrote *A Darker Ribbon: Breast Cancer, Women, and Their Doctors in the Twentieth Century*, which includes previously unpublished correspondence between pioneering environmentalist Rachel Carson and her surgeon, Dr. George Crile, Jr. Leopold is a member of the Women's Community Cancer Project in Cambridge, Massachusetts, and has written articles on breast cancer and women's health care for *The Nation*, *Self*, the *Chicago Tribune* and *Sojourner*.

Audre Lorde—black, lesbian, feminist, warrior, mother, poet, essayist, educator, activist, visionary—used the transforming events of her life to shape and empower her work. At her death from metastatic breast and liver cancer, which she battled for fourteen years, Lorde had published a wide body of work that included poetry, essays, memoir and lesbian-feminist theory.

Kelly Marbury is an ethical vegan born and raised in a small town in Pennsylvania. She graduated from Howard University with a degree in

Journalism/English. A natural technophile, Kelly cashed in her lifelong dream of winning the Pulitzer Prize in Journalism for a high-stress, claw-your-way-up-the-corporate-ladder career in computer sales. She enjoys playing golf, watching professional bicycle racing, and being in the company of her family and friends. Her goal in life is to be a mom.

Joan Nestle is a sixty-year-old Jewish femme woman who entered queer life in the working-class Greenwich Village butch-femme bars in the late 1950s. The author of *A Restricted Country* and *A Fragile Union* and editor of *The Persistent Desire: A Femme-Butch Reader*, she also co-founded the Lesbian Herstory Archives in New York City in 1973. She is grateful to every reader who has taken her word into her home.

Mona Oikawa is a Toronto-based writer and teacher. She is the co-author of *All Names Spoken* and her work has been published in *Countering the Myths: Lesbians Write About the Men in Their Lives*, *Privileging Positions: The Sites of Asian American Studies*, *The Very Inside* and other anthologies and journals. She is the co-editor of *Out Rage: Dykes and Bis Resist Homophobia* and *Resist!: Essays Against a Homophobic Culture*. Oikawa is an instructor at the Ontario Institute for Studies in Education at the University of Toronto. She is currently writing a book on the incarceration and forced displacement of Japanese Canadian women by the Canadian federal government in the 1940s.

Pat Parker died of breast cancer in 1989 at the age of forty-five. Poet Cheryl Clarke called Parker "a black, pre-integration, pre-baby boomer, post-McCarthy, transplanted Texan, lesbian-feminist San Franciscan and mother who knew how to kick ass in many arenas" in the introduction to the expanded edition of Parker's collected poems, *Movement in Black*. In 1977 Parker toured the U.S. performing her classic poem, "Movement in Black," with musicians Linda Tillery, Gwen Avery and Mary Watkins.

Paige Parvin is a writer for *Southern Voice* newspaper in Atlanta, Georgia. She holds a B.A. in English from the University of the South, Sewanee, and an M.A. in film studies from Emory University, with a focus on feminist and lesbian film.

Adrienne Rich was born in Baltimore, Maryland, in 1929. Since the selection of her first volume of poetry by W. H. Auden in 1951 for the Yale Series of Younger Poets, her work has continued to break new ground, moving from closed forms to a feminist poetics and a radical urban imagination and politics. Her books of poetry include *Collected Early Poems: 1950-1970*, *The Dream of a Common Language*, *Your Native Land, Your Life*, *Time's Power*, *An Atlas of the Difficult World*, *Dark Fields of the Republic* and *Midnight Salvage*. Prose works include *Of Woman Born: Motherhood as Experience and Institution; On Lies, Secrets, and Silence; Blood, Bread, and Poetry* and *What Is Found There: Notebooks on Poetry and Politics*. Rich's work has received many awards, including the Ruth Lilly Prize, the *Los Angeles Times* Book Award, the Lambda Literary Award, the Poet's Prize, the Lenore Marshall/Nation Award, a MacArthur Fellowship and the Dorothea Tanning Prize.

Ruthann Robson is on the board of www.sarcoma.net, a medical Web site providing information about the rare cancer of sarcoma. Her most recent collection of fiction is *The Struggle for Happiness*. She is also the author of *A/K/A, Eye of a Hurricane, Sappho Goes to Law School: Fragments in Lesbian Legal Theory* and *Lesbian (Out)Law: Survival under the Rule of Law*. Robson is a professor of law at the City University of New York School of Law.

Barbara Rosenblum, a creative sociologist, taught at Stanford University and Vermont College. She was widely published during her life in anthologies, journals and magazines as diverse as the *American Journal of Sociology*, the *San Francisco Chronicle* and *Sinister Wisdom*. Her book *Photographers at Work* was an early entry in the emerging field of the sociology of aesthetics. After a passionate career as a writer and teacher, Rosenblum died of breast cancer at age forty-four.

Teya Schaffer lives in Oakland, California. Her poetry and prose have appeared in the anthologies *Politics of the Heart: A Lesbian Parenting Anthology, The Tribe of Dina: A Jewish Women's Anthology* and *Women on Women: An Anthology of Lesbian Short Fiction*, as well as in various journals. Her first book, *A Ritual of Drowning: poems of love and mourning*, is dedicated to the memory of her spouse, Jackie Winnow.

Barbara Smith is the author of *The Truth That Never Hurts: Writings on Race, Gender and Freedom*. Books she has edited include *Home Girls: A Black Feminist Anthology* and (with Wilma Mankiller, Gwendolyn Mink, Marysa Navarro and Gloria Steinem) The *Reader's Companion to U.S. Women's History*.

Sandra Steingraber, Ph.D., received her doctorate in biology from the University of Michigan. The author of *Post-Diagnosis*, a volume of poetry and *Living Downstream: A Scientist's Personal Investigation of Cancer and the Environment*. She coauthored a report on ecology and human rights in Africa, *The Spoils of Famine*. She has been called "a poet with a knife" (*Sojourner*). She has taught biology for several years at Columbia College, Chicago, held visiting fellowships at the University of Illinois, Radcliffe College and Northeastern University and was appointed to serve on the National Action Plan on Breast Cancer, administered by the U.S. Department of Health and Human Services. As an ecologist, she has conducted field work in northern Minnesota, East Africa and Costa Rica. In 1997 Steingraber was named a Woman of the Year by *Ms.* magazine. In 1998 she received both the Will Solimene Award for Excellence in Medical Communications from the New England Chapter of the American Medical Writers

Association and the Jennifer Altman Foundation Award for "the inspiring and poetic use of science to elucidate the causes of cancer."

Jackie Winnow was a lesbian-feminist activist who brought her progressive politics (and love of cats) into all aspects of her life. She walked in the first women's liberation march held in New York City, did rape awareness work in Dade County, Florida, was an organizer of both the National Radical Feminist Conference and the 1982 San Francisco Jewish Feminist Conference. She worked as coordinator of the Lesbian/Gay & AIDS Unit of the San Francisco Human Rights Commission from 1980 to 1990. Diagnosed with cancer, Winnow responded by founding the Women's Cancer Resource Center in 1986—the first organization of its kind in the nation. Surivived by her spouse Teya Schaffer and Teya's son, Asher, Winnow died of metastatic breast cancer in 1991 at the age of forty-four with her work still unfinished.

Lisa D. Williamson is a writer and editor on the Philadelphia Main Line. Her fiction and nonfiction have appeared in numerous newspapers, magazines and anthologies. Williamson is a features writer for *Main Line Today* and sports editor for a local newspaper. She most loves interviewing and has interviewed luminaries from the literary and sports worlds as well as world- renowned chef George Perrier. She is currently at work on her second novel.

**Victoria A. Brownworth** is the author of eight books, including *Film Fatales: Independent Women Directors*, and the editor of nine, including *Restricted Access: Lesbians on Disability* and *Night Shade: Gothic Tales by Women*. She has been anthologized in numerous collections of fiction, nonfiction and poetry and has scripted four films. An award-winning journalist, her writing appears in numerous mainstream, queer and feminist publications, including the *Nation*, the *Village Voice*, *Ms.*, the *Philadelphia Inquirer*, the *Baltimore Sun*, *OUT* and *Girlfriends*. She has been a columnist for the *Philadelphia Inquirer*, the *Philadelphia Daily News*, the *Philadelphia Gay News*, the *Advocate*, *SPIN*, *Bay Area Reporter* and *Curve*. She lives in Philadelphia.

**The Mautner Project**, now celebrating its tenth anniversary of dedicated community service, is the nation's leading lesbian cancer organization. Through an innovative combination of local direct services and national outreach and education, the volunteer-driven organization provides support to lesbians with cancer, their partners and caregivers. Because risk reduction, early detection and proper care can greatly affect survival rates and quality of life, the Mautner Project educates and trains women who partner with women about all aspects of cancer. To break down the barriers preventing lesbians from getting the health care they need and deserve, the Mautner Project educates health care providers on the special concerns of lesbian clients and helps lesbians understand their rights as health care consumers.

Recognizing that cancer is not just a personal trauma but a public policy issue of tremendous importance, the Mautner Project plays a lead role in national advocacy on lesbian health issues, provides technical assistance to lesbian health projects throughout the country and coordinates the National Coalition of Feminist and Lesbian Cancer Projects. To receive help, information or referrals, or to make a contribution, please contact the Mautner Project at

The Mautner Project for Lesbians with Cancer
1707 L Street NW, Suite 500
Washington, DC 20036
Voice/TTY: 202-332-5536
Fax: 202-332-0662
email: mautner@mautnerproject.org
www.mautnerproject.org

## Selected Seal Press Titles

*Restricted Access: Lesbians on Disability* edited by Victoria A. Brownworth and Susan Raffo. $16.95, 1-58005-028-X. A book that explores the intersection of sexuality and disability and challenges the way America deals with difference.

*The Lesbian Health Book: Caring for Ourselves* edited by Jocelyn White, M.D., and Marissa C. Martínez. $18.95, 1-878067-31-1. This practical and readable book brings together a wide range of voices from the lesbian community, including doctors and other health care providers, women facing illness or life changes, health activists and many others.

*Lesbian Couples: A Guide to Creating Healthy Relationships* by D. Merilee Clunis and G. Dorsey Green. $16.95, 1-58005-41-7. A new edition of the highly acclaimed and popular guide for lesbians in couple relationships.

*The Black Women's Health Book: Speaking for Ourselves* edited by Evelyn C. White. $16.95, 1-878067-40-0. Features Alice Walker, bell hooks, Toni Morrison, Byllye Y. Avery, Audre Lorde, Faye Wattleton, Jewelle L. Gomez, Marian Wright Edelman and many others.

*Parting Company: Understanding the Loss of a Loved One: The Caregiver's Journey* by Cynthia Pearson and Margaret L. Stubbs. $18.95, 1-58005-019-0. A compassionate and revealing look at caregiving for the dying, including first-hand accounts of the dying process from a diverse group of caregivers as well as hospice and health care professionals.

*Ceremonies of the Heart: Celebrating Lesbian Unions* edited by Becky Butler. $16.95, 1-878067-87-7. Filled with ideas on creating unique rituals, this volume takes us into the lives of twenty-seven couples who have affirmed their relationships with weddings, holy unions and ceremonies of commitment.

*Chinese Medicine for Women: A Common Sense Approach* by Bronwyn Whitlocke. $12.95, 1-58005-018-2. An informative and accessible guide for women exploring alternative health remedies.

Seal Press publishes many books of fiction and nonfiction by women writers. If you are unable to obtain a Seal Press title from a bookstore, please order from us directly by calling 800-754-0271. Visit our website at www.sealpress.com.